Alzheimer's Challenged & Conquered?

Louis Blank

foulsham
LONDON • NEW YORK • TORONTO • SYDNEY

foulsham

The Publishing House,
Bennetts Close, Cippenham, Berks SL1 5AP, England

Neither the editors of W. Foulsham & Co. Limited
nor the authors or the publisher takes any
responsibility for any possible consequences from
any treatment, procedure, test, exercise, action or
application of medication or preparation by any
person reading or following the information in
this book. The publication of this book does not
constitute the practice of medicine, and this book
does not attempt to replace your Doctor. The
authors and publisher advise the reader to check
with a Doctor before administering any
medication or undertaking any course of treatment
or exercise.

Typeset in Great Britain by Typesetting Solutions, Slough, Berks.
Printed in Great Britain by St Edmundsbury Press Ltd
Bury St Edmunds, Suffolk.

Foreword by
Sir Cyril Smith, OBE

*

This book by Louis Blank is worth reading!

It is not difficult to read, and quite apart from Louis' experience, it contains much useful information. I have known Louis Blank for some time, and I know him to be an honourable man and an honest man.

Alzheimer's is NOT a pleasant illness – especially for the carer, who loves and watches and grieves. Can it be cured? – I know not. Nor does Louis claim it will work for everyone. He strongly believes he cured himself, and in this book he explains how.

I agree with his basic premise and I concede there is logic in his argument.

Anyway, buy the book. I recommend it. It's an interesting, easy read and it's educative. It may be helpful for while there is life, there is surely hope. Louis Blank, and his book, have my best wishes.

I would like to dedicate this book to my wife, but find the written word inadequate.

'With so many dimensions to my love for you,
How can I express it in just two?'

The author would like to thank his sister Valerie for proofreading this book. He would also like to thank the Arvon Centre, and particularly David Almond, for putting him on the right road.

* * *

Three doctors on three separate occasions diagnosed the author as having Alzheimer's disease. This is the story of how he set out to cure himself.

Both the author's wife and his daughter have written sections of the book due to his incapacity. They have indicated these sections in the story.

While the various authors may have changed some of the minor details, or mentioned them out of sequence to enable the story to flow more smoothly, all the material facts are true. The author may have altered the dialogue substantially, though not intentionally. Who can remember verbatim what was said some months ago? There may be other omissions due to memory loss caused by the disease itself.

Of course, everyone knows that there is, at present, no cure for Alzheimer's disease.
Everyone but the author.

Contents

*

Acknowledgements

*

This book would probably never have materialised without the help of Jean Jones and her team at Rochdale Library, and their unstinting help with my research.

Alzheimer's disease:
  'An incurable degenerative disease of unknown
cause affecting the central nervous system,
characterised by confusion, emotional instability, and
progressive mental deterioration.'
                                        Webster's Dictionary

Alzheimer's disease:
  'Something I used to have.'
                                        Louis Blank

Prologue

*

I slammed on my brakes and the Volvo 740 skidded to a halt just before it hit the garage door. Normally I would have sailed straight in but this time the up-and-over door had failed to rise when I had pressed the remote control button on my dashboard.

I was about to get out to open the door manually when the door suddenly swung upwards. It hit my front bumper and stopped. When I reversed the car the door rose, perhaps a little more slowly than normal, and I drove under the door and into the garage.

I examined the mechanism and it appeared to work perfectly once the door was open. It was only as I closed it from the outside that I saw the faint scratch marks where somebody had tried to pick the lock.

I glanced at the doors on the other garages in the basement block and saw that someone had managed to force several of them open. I re-adjusted the operating mechanism so that it ran as smoothly as before, and was glad to see that the security devices I had installed in the door had thwarted the thief.

I had made the remote control unit for the garage door several years ago when we had moved to this tower block. It is a simple device with two main parts. I cobbled up the first out of a car solenoid that releases a spring attached to the lock on the door, and the second is a remote control unit in my car. I built this out of some bits from the box of old electronic parts that I keep in my workshop. The security device is a little more complicated, but it was worth the time I spent on designing it. Thieves and vandals have attacked this garage block on numerous occasions, and the police seem powerless to do anything about it. Fortunately, no thief has yet succeeded in opening my garage door.

I was checking the control to make sure that it locked the garage securely when I gave a start as a voice behind me said, 'At least they didn't touch yours. They forced my door but fortunately my car wasn't in it. I think they pinched some of Don's old records though.'

I turned round and saw a stranger ruefully looking at the broken lock on the next garage. 'Someone did touch mine,' I replied, 'they tried to force the door but didn't manage it.'

I was about to explain about the security device I had built into the mechanism, but thought better of it. For all I knew, this could be the thief. He might not own the garage next door at all. I decided to humour him and see if he gave himself away. 'Was there anything else in your garage worth stealing?' I asked.

'Well, there's my old tool box and a jack and a couple of other bits and bobs in there, but they didn't touch any of it. Oh, and that reminds me . . .' He darted back in his garage and came out carrying a small red box with a couple of wires dangling from it. 'Here's your battery charger back,' he said, holding it out to me, 'If they'd got that, I suppose I'd have to buy you a new one. It did the job; I won't need it any more, the battery's fine now.'

I took the battery charger automatically as he handed it to me. I had never seen it before and wondered if he was confusing me with someone else. He did not look like a thief, and giving me this battery charger probably proved he was not. Unless it was a bluff, of course.

I was about to leave when he stopped me. 'Good news about Colin!'

'Eh?'

'I said it's good news about Colin; they say he'll be coming out next week.'

I wondered who Colin was, and where he was coming out from; prison perhaps? Maybe he was the stranger's crony.

I also wondered who that Don was that he referred to earlier. I did not know anyone by that name.

'Yes,' I said to humour him. 'That is good news. Well, I've got to go, see you again.' As I walked away, he called after me, 'Yes, see you, Louis. Look after yourself.'

'That's strange,' I thought, 'how does he know my name?'

I put it to the back of my mind for the moment, as I hurried to the lift of the tower block and just beat the closing doors. Three people entered at the ground floor, an elderly couple and a younger woman in her early thirties.

The man nodded as though he knew me so I nodded back. I was certain that I had never seem him before, but his wife seemed to know me also. This sort of thing had happened a lot lately, strangers nodding and smiling at me, and even addressing me by name.

'Good news about Colin,' the man said. 'You know, at one time I didn't think he'd make it, but they say he's nearly recovered.'

'Yes,' I said. I again wondered who Colin was. The man seemed to think that I should know all about it so I thought that I should humour him. 'I didn't think he'd make it either.' I wondered what Colin had tried to make.

The man's wife was talking to me now but I was not paying any attention to her. I was looking at the object I was carrying.

It was a small red box with two wires dangling from it. I knew what the box was for, and how it worked, but I could not think what it was called at the moment. The name escaped me.

It would come to me soon, it was on the tip of my er, my whatsit; you know, that wiggly thing in your mouth.

I must have picked this box up somewhere. If the lift had been empty, I could have put it on the floor and left it, but as it was, I coiled the wires up in my palm so they would not be conspicuous. If I had inadvertently stolen the box, I did not want anyone to notice until I could get rid of it. The young woman interrupted my thoughts as she said something to me. I pretended to ignore her, but she spoke louder so I looked up so as not to appear impolite.

She smiled a greeting at me. 'Hi,' she said, 'you been shopping?'

I guiltily tried to thrust the box behind me and mumbled something unintelligible as I looked down at the floor. I felt uncomfortable with the way she was staring at me.

When I was young, a lady would not speak to a strange man until someone introduced him to her. I peeked at her under my lowered brows, and with a start noticed that she was watching me in open-eyed frankness. She opened her mouth to say something, and I pretended to have a fit of coughing to forestall her. I did not want to make idle conversation with a young girl in a lift.

The couple got out at the ninth floor, and I was alone with the young woman. She was now looking at me openly, with a quizzical expression in her eyes.

Fortunately, I lived on the eleventh floor, but the lift seemed to crawl up forever before it finally came to rest and I could get out and away from her.

Keeping my eyes averted, I fled through the doors as soon as they opened and I sensed, even without seeing her, that she had got out as well. 'She must be visiting someone on my floor,' I thought. 'Strange, most of the people on this floor are still at work.' I put my key in the lock and opened the door. Suddenly, I was uncomfortably aware that the strange woman was right behind me. I tried to close the door but she put out her hand and held it open.

'W . . . what do you want?' I stammered.

'I want to come in, of course.'

Her brazen cheek took me aback. 'What do you mean, you "want to come in"?'

'I've come to visit you, Dad. What's the matter? You look as if you don't know me.'

'Ruth!' I gasped, and felt my head spinning. My God, it was true. There MUST be something wrong with me if I could not recognise my own daughter. It was not as if she had been away for several years. She lived only a couple of miles away and I saw her regularly.

Perhaps I should see the doctor after all.

CHAPTER ONE

Early Years to Early Retirement

*

I was born in Manchester in January 1937, just scraping in on the first hour of Aquarius, and we moved to London the following year.

My sister was born four years later on St Valentine's Day. After a great deal of imaginative thought, my parents named her 'Valerie'.

In the early 1940s, I was evacuated to Delamere, in Cheshire, for the duration of the war to escape the London blitz. By the time I returned to my family, they were living in Manchester, where we lived until I left school (Chorlton Park Secondary Modern) at the age of 15.

My family then moved to London and I got a job as a calculating machine mechanic with Monroe Calculators.

At 18, I began my National Service in the army. I joined the Rifle Brigade, a division of the Royal Green Jackets, and completed my ten weeks' basic training at Winchester.

I then went with my regiment to Kenya where there were problems with the Mau-Mau. At the end of 1956, the Rifle Brigade embarked for Malaya, and I was stationed at Kuala-Kuba-Bahru, a village near Kuala Lumpur, until my demob.

Back in 'Civvy Street' I worked in several shoe shops, first as a salesman, and later as a manager. For recreation, I joined a cycling club and went for weekend rides with them, and on Saturday evenings I went to the local dance hall.

It was at one of these dances that I noticed that a demure young girl sitting by a window seemed to have her eyes closed. Puzzled, I went up to see if she could possibly be asleep while the band was blaring out 'Rock Around the Clock'. I found that she was not asleep, but watching the dancers under her lowered eyelids. We chatted and she told me that her name was Sylvia.

As the music slowed to 'Moon River', she accepted my invitation to have the next foxtrot, my later invitation to take her home, and several months later, still another invitation to become my fiancée. (She told me later that the only reason she had allowed me to take her home was that she wanted a ride on my motorbike. Fortunately, she had not seen the motorbike before she agreed to let me take her home on it.)

This 'motorbike' (no serious motorcyclist would have dignified it by such a name) was a clapped-out 98cc James Comet that I had bought for £15 three weeks earlier. Although twice the capacity of the modern mopeds, it had nowhere near their performance.

According to the manufacturers, the Villiers engine produced two brake horsepower, but they must have been undernourished and sluggish horses as the bike would barely reach 25 mph on a long flat road.

The first night I took her home, the bike was far from impressive. I had never carried a pillion passenger before, and Sylvia lived at the top of Salter's Hill, a long 3-in-1 drag, in Upper Norwood. As we began riding up the base of the hill (flat out at about 15 mph), I changed down from top to bottom, the bike only having two gears.

It did not have a gear lever like the larger motorbikes, but a Sturmey-Archer lever on the handlebar similar to those on pedal cycles.

As the incline became steeper the bike slowed to a crawl.

'Paddle!' I shouted, demonstrating with my feet.

'What?' Sylia shouted back.

'Paddle with your feet or we'll stop. Never mind, it's too late.' I shouted as the engine stalled. 'We'll have to get off and push.'

We slogged and pushed the bike all the way up Salter's Hill, while I cursed its lack of power under my breath. It would not start at the top so we had to push it all the rest of the way to Sylvia's home.

There was an Ariel 'Square-Four' 1000 cc motorcycle combination parked outside her house, and when Sylvia told me that it belonged to her father, I cringed as he saw us pushing my 98 cc James up her path.

My first bike might have been puny, but I have since thanked God many times that I bought it. Sylvia did not mind helping me push the bike all the way to her house, but she probably would not have let me WALK her home.

In 1959 Sylia and I were married.

We went to Wales for our honeymoon, on another and larger motorcycle that broke down as we tried to ride up the Sugarloaf Mountain on it. We spent our wedding night at the side of the road as I tried to repair the bike and Sylvia did not utter one word of complaint as she held the torch for me. (Perhaps literally!)

We lived in a single room bed-sit until our daughter, Ruth, was born 14 months later and we then moved to a flat in Dulwich.

It was difficult to find somewhere to live at a reasonable rent in London, and we were overjoyed to find this place. It was part of the first floor of a private house and it consisted of a lounge, a kitchen and a bedroom.

With our own private kitchen, we really felt we had come up in the world, even though there was no hot water, just a single cold tap. The only heating was a small paraffin stove that caused the whole place to smell, and we had to constantly feed the electric meter to keep the light burning.

Our landlord lived below us, and we had to walk on tiptoe all the time as he was very sensitive to noise. I found this out on the first day when he came storming up to complain after I dropped a shoe on the floor instead of putting it down quietly. He told me that he had been sitting waiting for half an hour for the other shoe to fall!

Although we paid rent, he still regarded our flat as his property and kept a spare key so that he could inspect the place frequently. We always knew when he had been in while we were out, as we found his cigarette ends and neither Sylvia nor I smoke. However, we did not dare to say anything as, with a young baby to look after, we were lucky to have a place to live at all.

We remained there for two years and our son Michael was born in 1962.

On a Monday morning, two days before the birth, the shoe shop I worked for closed down and I was out of work.

I had bad stomach cramps on the Tuesday, and although Sylvia said that they were sympathy pains, I thought they were more likely to be the result of the stress of losing my job.

We were both wrong.

On Wednesday morning, the day Sylvia was due to go into hospital, the ambulance arrived. However, it was not for Sylvia – it was for me. I had appendicitis.

Sylvia stayed at home to wait for her ambulance, which came an hour later. However, before it arrived our landlord came up to tell her that he was giving us three days' notice to quit as he could not allow two children in the flat.

The upshot was that I was in one hospital and Sylvia in another and we had nowhere to live. I was out of work, we had a 2-year-old child and a new-born baby and in my pocket I had a letter from my bank manager asking me to call in to see him regarding an unauthorised overdraft.

Fortunately, Sylvia's parents agreed to look after Ruth until we both came out of hospital.

When we look back on this period, Sylvia and I both agree that it had an unexpected benefit that was to help us throughout our marriage. No matter how bad the hard times we have had since are, we always smile at each other and say, 'Well, we've pulled through worse, and at least it's not as bad as it was in 1962.'

I got a job with another shoe shop the day after I left hospital, and 12 months later the directors promoted me to manager. I left after a short while when a man, who I at first thought was a customer, offered me a position with a bespoke shop that supplied made-to-measure shoes.

They kept wood lasts of all their clients' feet and I numbered politicians and well-known entertainers among my customers. One day, a military type marched into the shop with a package under his arm. I asked him to sit down so that I could take his measurements, but he said there was no need for that and handed me the package. He was Douglas Bader, and the package contained a spare set of artificial legs.

Two years later, after working as a manager in a couple of other shops, I was the manager of the main branch of Dolcis in the Strand. It was one of the largest shoe shops in London, with 12 sales assistants on its staff. It seemed an exalted position but my salary was only £12 per week, and I seemed to be in a dead end as there did not appear to be any prospect of me rising any higher in the shoe trade.

Things really took a turn for the better in 1965. Sylvia noticed an advertisement by Nu-Swift Fire Protection for salesmen. I was reluctant to apply at first, as it was a 'commission-only' position, and I had a family to support. However, as Sylvia pointed out, this would just make me more determined to succeed.

I became a commission-only salesman and our standard of living immediately improved.

I worked for Nu-Swift for seven years, then joined Everest Double Glazing where I remained for another 12 years.

I then had a variety of sales jobs, usually as a salesman but occasionally as a sales manager.

Although my little James motorcycle disintegrated shortly after I met Sylvia (and was replaced by a succession of steadily newer and larger machines), a new and even smaller 'James' entered my life when Ruth got married and the following year (1979) gave birth to my first grandson.

Ruth has made steady progress in that direction, and I now have three more grandchildren, Sarah, Jacob and Esther.

Our lifestyle changed dramatically from the day I first worked on commission-only.

Take holidays for instance. Previously, we thought we were lucky to be able to go away for any sort of holiday. On our first one, we camped under a plastic sheet that I strung between two trees.

I told Sylvia that this was how we camped in the army under our ponchos, but she did not seem too keen on it, so the following year we saved up for a small tent.

We looked back on those camping holidays in future years, and they gave added zest to the cruises we now took round the Canary Islands or the holidays in exotic locations with Club Med.

It's strange that I should have begun to suffer from agoraphobia. If it had been claustrophobia, I would have understood. I previously preferred being in the open air than indoors. This applied as much to work as to my free time. Although I have been a sales manager and a company director, I never really liked these exalted positions. I would rather be out in the field as a salesman than work in an office.

I also regard it as a tremendous advantage that a commission-only salesman is paid on results. I have only had one pay rise in my life, and that was when I worked in a shoe shop before I went into the army. I went cap in hand to my boss and received a rise of five shillings (25p) per week.

Many commission-only salesmen earn more than some of the directors they work for, some more than the managing director. One year, my local newspaper published the salaries of MPs, and I noticed that I was earning slightly more than the prime minister.

As salesmen (unlike politicians) are paid only what they are worth, I think there is a moral there somewhere.

My life went smoothly for a few years. We bought a house in Rochdale, and soon moved to a larger detached one a few miles away in Shawclough, in the suburbs.

I spent a fair bit of money on this house, putting in a second bathroom, a fitted kitchen and a 26-foot-long patio door in the lounge. As I worked for Everest Double Glazing at the time, I got this patio door at a reduced price but the installation still cost a five-figure sum as it entailed a considerable amount of building work and an RSJ to support it.

I had a succession of fine cars, I enjoyed my work and was well paid for it, and life was sweet.

I should have known it could not last.

One day, I went to the vehicle licensing centre at Trafford House in Manchester to tax my car. In the entrance hall, there was the usual list of companies with offices in the building. Next to one of the names, Prestige Windows, there was a note stating that they were looking for salesmen. It seemed an unusual place for the offices of a double glazing company, so, out of curiousity, I took the lift to the third floor to have a look at them. It turned out to be the worst move of my life.

When the lift doors opened, I walked through two large double doors into one of the largest and most extravagantly sumptuous reception offices I have ever seen. There were enormous leather Chesterfields and armchairs scattered about, and the place gleamed with burr-walnut and mahogany. I walked across the seemingly never-ending carpet to the girl smiling at me from behind the reception desk. She handed me an application form which I completed.

Although I had no intention of changing jobs when I entered the building, the opulent surroundings had had the desired effect and I became an enthusiastic salesman for Prestige Windows the following week.

I soon began to realise that there was something odd about the firm. For one thing, the enormous reception area was purely for show. A door at the back led to half a dozen poky offices, where about 30 people worked in very cramped conditions. Prestige Windows was part of a larger company called the Plygrange Group. They sold a wide variety of home improvements, from loft insulation to central heating systems, and all the offices of the firm were in these few small rooms.

I put my misgivings to one side because the money was good and I got on well with Derek, the sales manager, who seemed an honest enough chap.

However, Derek left a few weeks after I joined, and the directors offered me his job. Like a fool, I took it.

I arrived at work one morning to find the place vacant. The directors had used the firm solely to build up a line of credit, and then liquidated everything and fled the country.

I got another job with a double glazing firm in Stockport, and thought that was the end of it. About six months later, I opened a letter from my accountant telling me that I was due for a small tax rebate as I had overpaid the previous year. A couple of weeks later, I received a cheque from the Inland Revenue for £145.

The following month, I received a tax demand for £178 652.

I remembered joking about it with Sylvia. It was such an unbelievable amount that we knew it must be a computer error.

Unfortunately, it was not.

I was told later that the Plygrange directors were working a tax fiddle and claimed to be employing over 200 salesmen for Prestige Windows. They apparently received a cash incentive for every extra person they employed. As a sales manager, I had received an override of 2.5 per cent of all the salesmen's commissions, and the tax demand was based on the tax inspector's estimate of the commission for the sales force.

I protested that we had never employed more than seven salesmen, but the directors had taken the books and accounts with them, and I had no way of proving that I did not employ the fictitious number they claimed.

Without any records it's still an easy thing to prove that you DO employ a number of people. You just have to give their names and addresses. It's a very different matter to prove that you did NOT employ a group of nameless people.

I appealed and lost when my accountant would not become involved in it because there were no books or other records with which he could draw up a balance sheet.

I appealed again, and lost once more, and this time had considerable legal fees to pay.

I had the option of further appeals, right up to the House of Lords, but not being eligible for legal aid meant that the rapidly rising costs would soon be as horrendous as the tax assessment.

The outcome was that the Inland Revenue took my house, and we went to live in a council flat.

They also took a pension that I was hoping to retire on, and surrendered it for its cash value. They sold the house for less than half what it was worth, together with most of our possessions, but left me my Mercedes as a 'tool of my trade'.

Shortly after that I developed an ulcer and began taking Aludrox, an antacid remedy containing aluminium.

I traded in the Mercedes against a Volvo to raise a bit of cash to live on, and got a job with another window company.

As the house and other items had realised only half of the tax demand and legal costs, the Inland Revenue took part of my commission cheque each week. As in the early days, we were again having to scrimp and scrape, and I began carrying bottles of Aludrox in the glove compartment of my car. Sylvia wanted me to see the doctor, but I suspected that he would recommend an operation, and I could not afford the time off work.

I worked harder than ever, and just took a swig from the Aludrox bottle whenever I needed it to keep me going.

My new firm had a high turnover of salesmen as they kept finding reasons for not paying commission cheques. Each week there was a different excuse, and each salesman had to argue over his pay cheque before the reluctant director released it.

After 12 months of arguing about my commission, I left and took them to court for an outstanding balance of £1254. I won the case, but gained nothing other than the satisfaction of winning. My barrister did not bother to apply for costs, and so the judge did not make an order about them.

When I asked my solicitor when I would be getting my money, he said that my legal costs were £1323 and could I please forward him the balance of £69 by return.

Things improved in November 1987 when I left the firm I was with to join Wilson & Glick Kitchens Ltd. This proved to be the sort of job I had always been seeking. However, I still had bad stomach pains and continued to take Aludrox.

The firm was formed only two weeks before I joined it by three partners, Harvey Wilson (of whom more later), Martin Glick and Alan Sheldon. It was a company that they had created to supply quality kitchens at a realistic price. They only had one salesman so far, and I welcomed the challenge of helping to get a new firm off the ground.

Their product was of a good quality and at a realistic price. As with my previous firms, they paid me on a commission-only basis and I earned a good living. The firm expanded rapidly and after six months they had taken on ten more salesmen.

I enjoyed my work and, apart from the tax burden, the only other problem I had was with an arthritic hip.

I had been waiting for a hip replacement for several years, but when I first went to see a specialist he was reluctant to carry out the operation because he considered that I was too young. As the life expectancy of an artificial hip is about ten years, surgeons prefer patients in their seventies or older. There is then only a small chance that the hip replacement will fail, and itself require replacing after a few years. This is not just on economic grounds. Apparently, it is much more difficult to replace a hip for the second or subsequent time than it is initially.

The fairly gruesome details are as follows . . . (sensitive readers may wish to skip the next few paragraphs):

Dr Charnley of Wrightington Hospital, near Wigan in Lancashire, developed the modern hip replacement. It superseded an older version that surgeons wired to the outside of the femur rather like a splint. The modern one is a vast improvement. It consists of a plastic cup, which works in conjunction with a one-piece chrome-molybdenum ball and rod as is shown here. The existing hip joint is sawn off, then the remaining bone has the marrow in its centre drilled out so that it forms a tube into which the surgeons insert a chrome rod. They then fix this permanently in place with an epoxy adhesive.

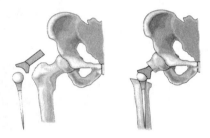

The problem is that there is no solvent for this adhesive, or rather no solvent that would be safe to use. This means that if the replacement hip needs renewing several years later, the surgeon has to laboriously chip away the adhesive.

Surgeons are reluctant to do this as it is a far longer and more involved operation than drilling the bone in the first place.

However, my hip had worsened over the years until Mr Knott, the main orthopaedic surgeon at Rochdale Infirmary, eventually put me on his list.

At the beginning of May 1988, I received a postcard telling me to report to Rochdale Infirmary on the 14th to have a hip replacement the following day.

I told Martin Glick that I would need some time off work, and that it would probably be at least three months, and his reaction surprised me.

Having been a commission-only salesman for many years, I was used to the prevalent attitude in the profession. There is no such thing as holiday or sick pay; if you do not sell, you do not eat. I had not met anyone like Martin in it previously.

'So they're going to operate at last. Good, you shouldn't have to wait for something like that,' he replied when I told him. 'Are you worried about it?'

'Well, I suppose I am a bit. It's a routine operation, but still fairly major.'

'I'm not just talking about the operation itself, are you worried about anything else?'

'Should I be? I suppose you'll keep my job open for me?'

'That goes without saying. Anything else?'

'Well, I suppose things will be a bit tricky financially until I get back to work, but we'll manage somehow.'

'I thought so!' replied Martin. 'Now you might still worry about the operation itself, but that'll be over within a couple of days. As for financial worries, I don't want you to be bothered with them. It doesn't matter whether you're off for three months or three years. You've got £400 a week coming in until you're able to get back to us.'

I just could not believe it. He was going to advance me £400 a week out of future commissions for an indefinite period. I had never known anything like that in direct sales before, particularly with a salesman who had only been with the firm for a few months.

I thought about it for a moment. It was an astoundingly generous offer, but perhaps too generous. If I accepted, I would owe the firm £5000 or more when I resumed work. Without the travelling and other expenses my job entailed, Sylvia and I would be able to manage on far less than £400 a week while I was off work.

The less I borrowed, the less I would have to repay.

I shook Martin's hand. 'That's very good of you, boss, but I think I can manage on less than that while I'm off work. Call it £200 a week and you've got yourself a deal.'

The operation went smoothly, without any complications. It was a source of discomfort more than anything else. I had to lie flat on my back for the following week, with my legs in two open-topped padded boxes. With their quilted lining and stout wooden sides, they looked just like open coffins.

Watson Ward at Rochdale Infirmary was a mixed ward with men down one side and ladies down the other. The morning after my operation, I was awakened by a voice wailing, 'Where am I?' There was a torrent of abuse from a couple of men farther down the ward, then a nurse came in to soothe the elderly lady opposite me. As soon as she left, the lady cried out again, 'Where am I?'

Thinking that perhaps she had awakened from an operation and could not get her bearings, I called out, 'You're in Rochdale Infirmary.'

'It's no good telling her that, she's a loony,' the man at the end shouted.

The lady called out the same question at regular intervals, and took no notice of any remarks or answers. The first thing I did when they allowed me to get up for a few minutes was to hobble across to her.

I had a large card (from the back of a get well card) and wrote on it in felt tip, 'You are in Rochdale Hospital, you will soon be better and the nurses will look after you.'

I thought that this might reassure her, but it made no difference, she still kept calling out in her lost voice.

I asked the doctor about her later and he told me she was suffering from Alzheimer's disease. I had already guessed as much. My mother was in a similar condition shortly before she died.

The boredom and discomfort made the ten days of enforced bed rest seem like a month. I could not even read for more than a few minutes. Lying flat on my back meant I had to hold a book or paper up at such an angle that my arms soon ached. The knowledge that I would not be able to work for a further three months depressed me. Yes, a real misery-guts, that's what I was.

Until one morning, utterly bored, I idly reached for the headphones above my bed and listened to the music for a while. When the disc jockey came on, my boredom vanished. It was David Langer, the sales director of Wilson & Glick.

I remembered him telling me that he worked for hospital radio in his spare time, but it was just something mentioned in passing, and I forgot about it soon afterwards. Now here he was, laughing and joking between the records. It was like listening to a voice from home.

I left hospital a fortnight after my operation, and for a week or so could only hobble about on two sticks. I improved rapidly, and three months to the day after I left work, I returned.

One evening, on the way home from a customer, I called at David's house in Prestwich to give him the order I had just obtained.

He had a beautiful house that was on my route home, and if I took the order to him there, I would not need to go into the office the following day.

While we were chatting, I mentioned about hearing him on the radio in hospital, and he took me into the cellar from which he broadcasts. Until then, I thought he performed as a disc jockey as a hobby, but when I saw the equipment in his cellar, I realised that this was a major obsession with him. He had it laid out like a miniature recording studio to a very professional standard. I realised that he must regard the hospital radio as his main passion, and Wilson & Glick was the hobby.

Are you listening, Martin Glick?

When I had been back at work for a few weeks, I mentioned something to Sylvia that had been puzzling me.

'Have you noticed something, dear?'

'No, what's that?'

'My commission cheques. I thought they would have started taking a bit off each week for what I owe them, but they're still paying me the full amount. I'd better mention it, we don't want the debt hanging over our heads for ever.'

'Yes, but perhaps they are just waiting till you get back on your feet properly. I should give it another couple of weeks or so, and if they haven't taken any off by then, have a word with Mr Glick.'

The following month I spoke to Martin, as I had still not had any deductions from my commission.

'Hi, boss, got a minute?'

'Sure, come into my office.'

I followed him in and closed the door behind me. He had told me not to mention anything to the other sales staff about the money I was receiving or, as he put it, 'They'll all be queuing up for bloody hip replacements.'

'I was just wondering', I began, 'when you're going to start taking the money out of my commission cheques to pay back what I owe you?'

'Oh, and what do you owe us?' he asked.

'You know, the £200 a week you advanced me all the time I was off work.'

'Oh that! That wasn't an advance. That was just from the firm to you as a gesture of our esteem.'

'You mean I don't have to pay it back?'

'No, of course not. Now get your bloody backside out of here. You should be out there flaming selling, not pestering me with stupid questions.'

'Right, boss', I said as I left. I paused and turned in the doorway. 'Er, Martin?'

'Yes?'

'As I don't have to pay it back, can we review it and backdate it?'

'What do you mean, review it?'

'Well, I think I'll accept your original offer of £400 a week!'

I left hurriedly as he picked up a heavy book to throw at me.

The year after my hip replacement, I had another couple of weeks in hospital, this time for a slipped disc.

I can trace my back trouble to the days when I worked for Nu-Swift Fire Protection, as a salesman and service engineer. I reached up to remove a 2 gallon (later upgraded to 10 litres) water extinguisher off a customer's wall. For some reason, this was hanging on a bracket far above the recommended height of 2 metres from the floor. As I lifted the extinguisher down, it twisted in my arms and began to drop behind me.

There is an old saying about not catching falling objects, 'Never chase a falling knife, or a runaway wife; they're both sharp!'

I did not heed this adage and, instead of letting the fire extinguisher drop, I retained my grip on it and twisted my back. I believe this is the cause of the backache I have had over the years.

Mr Knott, the surgeon who did my hip replacement, performed a laminectomy, which involved removing the old disc and replacing it with one made of nylon. This completely cured the problem; I have never had the slightest twinge since then, and I would recommend the operation to anyone who needs it.

One thing I would not recommend though is the lumbar puncture they did a couple of days before they operated. This caused the most agonising pain I had ever experienced. It lasted only for a minute or two but seemed to go on for hours. Unfortunately, that was not the end of it. I got cramps in the middle of the night that caused me to keep bending double and straightening again.

It was agony to move my back at all, yet here I was doubling up uncontrollably with cramp. After each spasm, I would wait for the pain to subside a little, then gingerly lower myself back down on the bed and wait for the next one. I tried clutching the sides of the mattress to prevent myself from jerking upright, but this had no effect: I still shot upright out of control. The more I tried to remain flat to ease the pain, the more violently I doubled up as the cramps hit me. Even before I had the lumbar puncture it was agony to bend my back, and now I was bending and straightening with cramps against my will.

I think I would almost rather watch a party political broadcast on television than go through that lot again.

Apart from the agony following the lumbar puncture, I thought that the whole operation went smoothly. It was not until several months after I had returned home that Sylvia told me the full story. On the afternoon of my operation, I was still in the theatre at the time the sister had told her I was due back on the ward. When I had still not returned to the ward an hour later, Sylvia tried to contact a doctor to see how I was. He had no news then, and neither had the sister half an hour later.

Eventually, the sister told Sylvia that she would not be able to see me until the following day as I was in a critical condition. Apparently I had stopped breathing during the operation and they had had to resusitate me. Later a nurse confided to Sylvia, 'At one time, we thought we'd lost him.' I now wonder how long my brain was without oxygen during this episode, and whether it could have any bearing on my present condition.

*   *   *

On the 15th of June 1992 Martin Glick called a meeting in the sales office. We all knew that it was bad news. Twelve months had passed since Harvey Wilson, the senior partner, had left, since when the company had begun a slow decline. Recently there had been several indications that all was not well with the firm. We thought that Martin might have been going to tell us that owing to the financial situation he was going to delay payment of our annual bonus.

Martin paid these bonuses to all salesmen who achieved a sales target. Out of the present sales force of about 80 only ten of us had reached this target, so most of the salesmen at the meeting thought it did not concern them.

They were wrong.

Martin had to stop to wipe his eyes as he told us that the firm was in a far worse state than we had realised and was going into liquidation. This came as a tremendous blow to me. I had been happier working for Wilson & Glick than any previous firm and, at 55, I felt that I might have difficulty getting another job.

Also not only had Sylvia and I been counting on my £6000 bonus, we had practically spent it in advance.

Two days later, there was a particularly harrowing meeting in the sales office, when the receivers took the firm out of Martin's control. Not surprisingly, Martin broke down in tears as they began to dismantle the firm he had striven so hard to build.

There is a strange aspect about my time with Wilson & Glick that I did not find out until after they went into liquidation.

Of the three partners, Martin Glick, the managing director, was the one I came into contact with most frequently. Alan Sheldon was on the administration side, and I rarely saw Harvey Wilson, the chairman. As I mentioned, he left the company about a year before it folded. I later found out that he set up a new firm called Mr Wilson's Kitchens.

Several months after the firm's collapse, my sister Valerie (who lives in Poole, near Bournemouth) came to visit me. She intended to pop in to see one of our cousins on the way. As she was late, I telephone Joyce, my cousin whom I had lost contact with for several years until Valerie gave me her phone number, to see if she was still there. She told me Valerie had left about an hour before. During our conversation, she asked me what I was doing these days.

'I'm selling kitchens,' I told her, 'have been doing for a few years, but just changed firms because the old one has collapsed.'

'Oh, I'm sorry to hear that. I hope you do well in your new one. Funny that, you being in kitchens as well.'

'Oh, what do you mean, "as well"? As well as what?'

'As well as your cousin Harvey; he's in kitchens too.'

'Really, I didn't even know I had a cousin Harvey. Who is he?'

'He's my son.'

'Oh, well I've never met him. I knew your parents, Uncle Jack and Aunt Milly, but we moved down to London before you got married.'

'So you never met your cousin Harvey. Not met any of the Wilson's side of the family then?'

'Nope, never did. Wait a minute, did you say Wilson. Good grief, I'm slow. I didn't even know your married name was Wilson. Tell me it's not."

'Yes, it is. Something wrong?'

'No. Only that I've been working for Harvey Wilson for four years and neither of us knew we were related.'

*   *   *

Perhaps the sudden collapse of Wilson & Glick could have contributed to my condition. However, a few weeks later, I received a phone call from Martin.

He sounded his old cheerful self. With the help of David Langer, the sales director of Wilson & Glick, and three other of his old employees, he was starting a new company called Marshall Blake Kitchens.

'Would you like to join me as my one and only salesman?' he asked.

I told him that I would. I stayed with him as his new firm gradually expanded.

When I first joined Marshall Blake, my sales performance was at its peak. This was because I was the only member of the sales force, and was conscious that the future of the company depended on me. Occasionally, if I had more calls than I could handle, Martin would deal with the excess, and made one or two sales. (All right, Martin, perhaps three or four.) Even Keith Bradburn, a former surveyor of Wilson & Glick who was a director of the new company, went to visit a customer on occasion, but I was responsible for 90 per cent of the business.

However, as the firm expanded and the pressure eased off, my sales started to drop. They continued to fall, and although I was still earning a reasonable living, I realised that there was something drastically wrong. I left several customers in the middle of a sale by saying that I had given them enough to think about for one evening, and would make an appointment in a few days when they had talked it over. The reality was that I just could not concentrate on the job for more than an hour or so. The paperwork became very difficult to do, and if the customer required finance, which entailed much form filling, I said that I had no documents with me and would return with them another day. This was because I could no longer fill in a finance form, and I lost several sales because of it. It became increasingly difficult to work, until on the 15th of May 1993, I had to retire due to illness. I have recently learned that Martin has also left Marshall Blake Kitchens and is now with a stationery firm. I wish him all the best; his kind is very rare.

* * *

As I have always been a workaholic, the thought of retiring terrified me at first. My father continued to run a small accounting practice until the day of his death, at the age of 86. Although I had never given it much thought, I had always imagined that I would remain working as long. Three years ago, my old school-mate and lifelong friend, Peter Hewitt, retired. He left a good job as an engineer for an insurance company that he seemed to enjoy. I asked him about it, and he told me that he was 'retiring to play golf'. I shook my head and told him that I would be working into old age, because selling was a way of life to me, and I could not imagine doing anything else. How wrong I was.

My sudden retirement meant there would be a problem about money. Years ago, I had taken out an insurance policy that I could convert to a pension scheme when I retired. Unfortunately, the salesman had persuaded me to opt for a policy that I could surrender for a cash sum in an emergency. I had thought that this was a prudent move, but it proved to be otherwise. The Inland Revenue confiscated it and cashed it in, whereas if I had taken out a policy that I could not cash in until my retirement, it would have been safe and would also have had a higher yield.

I had three other policies of the latter type, but they were very small, and the total amount payable would be far less per year than I was earning per week as a salesman.

Sylvia told me, 'Not to worry, we'll manage somehow dear, we always do', and seemed so confident about it that I left it to her. She claimed and received a disability living allowance for me, and eventually a carer's allowance for her. This was supplemented by income support from the DHSS. At one time, I would have run a mile rather than accept income support or the like. However, I now felt that I had paid so much more than my fair share to the Inland Revenue that I was probably supporting half the unemployed population of Lancashire.

Before my illness, I would have taken complete control of the situation, and would probably have sat down and worked out a budget to suit our finances.

Now I just accepted Sylvia's word that we would manage and. left her to cope.

CHAPTER TWO

Lost Memories

(dedicated to all Alzheimer's disease sufferers)

✳

The present is but an instant,
  the future's not yet here,
'Tis the past, the past, that moulds us,
  and holds our memories dear.
Our memories of past events,
  of Loves, and Laughs, and Sorrows,
Of sharing plans from yesteryear,
  and hopes for new tomorrows.

Memories of years long gone,
  and of more recent days,
Make us what we are today,
  and guide our present ways.
Should our memory e're be lost,
  through accident or ill-health,
There could be no tragedy greater than,
  to lose such precious wealth.

The man, or woman, with such a loss,
  has been stricken such a blow,
When asked who, or what, or where they are,
  To have to answer 'I don't know'.

'i don't know where i'm going,
And i don't know where i've been,
i don't know what i've just been told,
    Or what i have just seen,
But there's one thing that i do know,
    As you may have guessed,
    i do know that i don't know.
    When i don't my mind will rest'

O cruel fate to strike one so,
    and to have added yet,
A new poignant meaning to the words,
    'Lest we forget'.

Sylvia had been trying to persuade me to visit the doctor for several months, but I kept refusing to go. When my daughter told her how I failed to recognise her in the lift, Sylvia decided that it had gone on long enough. 'I'm sorry, but you're going to see the doctor if I have to drag you there myself. Ruth, ring the surgery please, the number's on the pad.'

Ruth picked up the phone to make an appointment, but hung up when the receptionist asked her if she could phone back in the morning because it was after hours and she was just leaving.

'Well, I'll ring them to make an appointment first thing in the morning,' Sylvia said. 'You've really got to see him; you're becoming so forgetful, there must be something wrong.'

'I'm not forgetful,' I mumbled. 'It's just that I've got a lot on my mind. Someone tried to break into my garage.'

'Yours as well! I was talking to Don earlier and he told me they pinched some of his records. He's very upset because some of them are his original recordings and there are no other copies. Did they manage to get into YOUR garage?'

'No, but they did get in one or two others. Who's Don?'

She looked at me. 'You know. Don; from the floor below. Don Estelle. *"It ain't half hot, Mum"*. Surely you remember Don?'

'Oh yes, of course. Don. Of course, I remember him.' I lied. I could not recall any Don, but she seemed to think I should so I decided to humour her. Idle conversation rarely seemed to make sense to me these days.

Why did she call me 'Mum' and why was she talking about it being hot in the middle of winter? I felt the radiator, but it was no warmer than usual.

'But you didn't even recognise ME!' Ruth interrupted my thoughts. She seemed very upset.

'Well, that's nothing to do with my memory. You know how short-sighted I am without my glasses.'

'But you've got your glases on!'

I lifted my hand and touched them. 'Oh yes, well I must have put them on when I came in.'

'No, you didn't, you were wearing them all the time.'

Good grief, this was turning into an interrogation! They would be shining a spotlight into my eyes and wiring me up to a lie detector any minute. I snapped at Ruth to end the conversation. 'Well, you know how dark it is in the lift. Anyway, I don't want to talk about it any more. I've got things to do.'

I stormed out of the room and into my den where I picked up a book and pretended to read it in case anyone came in after me.

I sat deep in thought. I could not visit the doctor in case he stopped me from driving. As a sales representative, driving was a necessity. At 55 I would find difficulty in getting another job. Apart from illness and holidays,

I had never been out of work in my life, and dreaded the thought of it now. It was not just for financial reasons. Although things would be difficult, I knew we would manage somehow.

The thought of being idle was a different matter. As a workaholic, the prospect of being unemployed horrified me.

Thankfully, neither Sylvia nor Ruth mentioned the subject again that day.

Next morning at breakfast, I grimaced as I drank my orange juice.

'What's the matter, dear?' asked Sylvia, taking a sip of hers. 'It's the usual brand, and mine tastes all right.'

'No, the juice is okay. Just got a twinge of toothache, that's all."

I immediately realised that I had said the wrong thing as Sylvia replied, 'Do you want me to make you an appointment with the dentist?'

'No, it's all right now; ouch!' It definitely was not all right.

I finished my breakfast, holding my head on one side so that nothing would set my tooth off again, and Sylvia phoned the surgery as soon as they opened. I could hear her voice on the phone through the open door of my den. I was half-hoping that they would not be able to fit me in today. I was out of luck.

'Yes, the name's Blank,' I heard her say. 'Louis Brian . . . Let me see, about 12 months ago I think . . . Yes . . . came on this morning at breakfast . . . Yes please, 11 o'clock; I'll tell him. Thank you.'

She came into my den. 'I've made you an appointment for 11. Do you want me to come with you?'

'Of course not. I'm quite capable of going to the dentist on my own.'

'Yes, of course you are dear. It's just that you have been acting a bit strange lately. I just wondered if you would like some company.'

'I've not been acting strange at all. Just had a lot on my mind, that's all. Anyway if I'm going to finish this before I go, I'd better get on with it.' I bent down to the small electric motor I was rewiring, and Sylvia took the hint and left me to it. I suppose I half-hoped we would both forget all about it, but with things like dental appointments, Sylvia is infallible. At half past ten, she came in with my coat and waved me goodbye.

✳   ✳   ✳

'Blank?' the receptionist said in a puzzled voice. 'I don't seem to have you down. When was this appointment made?'

'My wife phoned you this morning. But never mind, if you've not got me down, I'll come back another day.'

'Just a minute,' she said, 'I'll just check when you were last here, and make you another appointment.' She studied her computer screen and logged on to my records. 'Hmm, I see it's nearly three years since you were here last.'

'As long as that?' I said in surprise.

'Yes, it is Louis Brian Blank of. . .' She read out my address and I confirmed that we were talking about the same person.

'Well, how would next . . .' she began, then paused and looked up from the screen. 'Oh, I see we can fit you in this morning. We've had a cancellation.' My heart sank. My toothache had gone and I wanted to forget the whole business. However, she had a vacant appointment slot in a quarter of an hour, and so I reluctantly decided to wait. I looked at my watch. If she did not call my name within 15 minutes, I would tell her I could not stay any longer and let Sylvia make me an appointment for another day. Preferably in ten years' time.

There were several other people in the waiting room. Among them was a lady with her 6- or 7-year-old daughter, and an elderly couple talking quietly together near the window. A business man, who kept looking at his watch and muttering to himself, sat next to the only vacant seat. I sat down and, as I did not want to appear nervous, I picked up the nearest magazine and pretended to read it. I felt a nudge in my ribs and turned to the business man.

'You can wait forever in these places.' He obviously wanted to strike up a conversation to take his mind off other matters.

'Yes', I said, 'but I can't wait too long. If they don't see me in a few minutes, I'm going to have to come back another time.'

'Me too', he replied glumly.

I thought he might be a bit nervous, so decided to try to cheer him up a bit. 'You know what? I'm nearly 60 and I've got all my own teeth.'

'Really,' he replied, as he again looked at his watch.

'Yes,' I laughed, 'I finished paying for them last week!'

He looked at me and mumbled something, picked up the nearest magazine and apparently found something fascinating in one of the articles. After ten minutes, I put down my magazine. It was not worth waiting the remaining five minutes. They were obviously far too busy to see me today. I stood up and was about to leave when the receptionist looked up and spoke.

'Will you go in now, Mr Blank? First door on the left down the corridor. Mr Jackson is waiting for you.'

I did not remember Mr Jackson, but he seemed to know me. 'Please take a seat, Mr Blank,' he said, indicating an ominous black leather chair.

'I'll be with you in a moment. It's quite a while since we've seen you here. Now then, let's see if there is any deterioration.'

I sat in the chair and he began the treatment by shining a small torch in my eyes. I had heard somewhere about this technique of hypnotism to take away pain, but assumed that they had to ask your permission first.

However, I just wanted to get it all over with so did not make any objections.

He shone the torch into both eyes, and when he asked me if I could see the small red dot on the wall in front of me, everything clicked into place.

So that was the reason they had so many spectacle frames on the walls!

I did not want the optician to think that I was an idiot, so I let him continue with the full treatment.

I then had to go through the rigmarole of choosing new frames.

'Your glasses will be ready by Thursday, or Friday at the latest. We'll telephone you at home; I've got the number,' the receptionist called after me as I left.

When I got home Sylvia called out from the kitchen.

'Where on earth have you been? The dentist phoned to ask where you were, and I told him you set out in plenty of time. I just phoned him back a few moments ago, and he says you have not been at all. Whatever happened?'

'Oh,' I said, 'I got a bit of grit in my eye on the way there, and as I was passing the opticians, I popped in to see if they could get it out. They made me wait while they did a full eye examination, and then told me I needed new glasses. They'll be ready on Thursday or Friday.'

'Talk about high pressure selling!' Sylvia said. 'I'll just phone them and give them a piece of my mind.'

'No, don't do that,' I said.

'If they say I need new glasses, then I probably do. They gave me a very thorough examination. That's why I didn't have time to go to the dentist.'

'Oh, all right,' Sylvia said. 'We'll get the glasses this time, but we'll find another optician in future. I don't think it's ethical dragging people in off the street like that.'

Despite many similar incidents, I made up my mind that I was not ill; I told myself that the lapses of memory were due to preoccupation. As for not recognising my daughter, I thought that perhaps she had a new hairstyle or something.

As a salesman, my life has always been full of pressure, and I used to thrive on it. I found the job exhilarating. The tremendous highs, with the adrenaline coursing through my veins on making a sale that others might not have managed, more than made up for the dismal lows when I had not sold anything for a few days. Lately, however, the pressure began to have an effect on me. Although some of this pressure was self-induced, a great deal of it was external. Some of it was created deliberately by the firm.

An example of this is the way appointments were issued. As it was considered essential that both husband and wife should be at home when the salesman called, the Monday to Friday appointments were made for the evening. A member of the office staff would begin ringing the customers after 5.30 p.m. to confirm that both partners would be at home.

As each appointment was confirmed, he would ring the relevant salesperson and pass on the time of the appointment and the name and address of the customer.

I was usually on tenterhooks awaiting my evening telephone call, as I then had the minimum time to sort out the relevant maps, plan my route, and drive to the address that was usually about a hundred miles or so away.

I often wondered why there were no customers living near Manchester who were interested in kitchens, until one day I found out the reason. I had an appointment in Newcastle-upon-Tyne, and the following day, I telephoned the salesgirl who lived in Newcastle about another matter and mentioned that I had called on a customer near her the previous evening. When she told me that she had been given an appointment for the previous evening in Middleton, only a few miles from my home, I decided to ask David Langer, the sales director, why the appointments were not issued to the nearest salesman.

I had to call in the office that morning anyway, so went in to see him. He told me that the appointments were issued to the farthest salesperson deliberately. He explained his philosophy. If salespersons had to make an investment in time and petrol of driving a considerable distance to see a customer, they would be more determined to make a sale than if they had merely popped round the corner. I suppose that it made a weird sort of sense, if you discounted the fact that a sale would be more likely if a salesperson arrived fresh rather than tired from a long drive. The firm might also have reconsidered the philosophy if they had been paying for the petrol.

As the pressure started getting to me, I began dreading the evening phone calls, and hoping that this evening I would NOT have an appointment. This was in total contrast to the way I used to feel. The thought of a two-hour drive in the evening, spending three or four hours with a customer, and then driving home in the early hours of the morning made me cringe. I dreaded this homeward journey when I was tired. Several years ago, I had worked for Vogel Kitchens, when a colleague of mine, Duncan Wyllie, died in a motorway accident. There were no other vehicles involved; he simply drove into a bridge support. The coroner's statement said that the road surface was dry, there were no skid marks, and he could only assume that Duncan had fallen asleep at the wheel.

Lately, I had often found myself nodding off at the wheel. I always pulled off at the next motorway exit and had a 15-minute nap, but sometimes the next exit was several miles away and it became increasingly difficult to concentrate. I almost considered giving up my life as a salesman and seeking an office job.

An accident took the decision out of my hands a few days later. I was on my way home after visiting a customer in Northumberland.

My 'conversion rate' (that is, sales to calls), used to be fairly high, but it seemed to have dropped lately. I did not get an order this evening, and left about 11.30 p.m.

It was now about 1.30 a.m., raining heavily, and I felt tired and depressed. Driving used to be a pleasure, but lately it had become less so. Sometimes I found it quite a strain, and I frequently had to stop to check the road atlas when I forgot the route. Also the homeward journey, no matter what the distance, always seemed far longer and more depressing on the days when I did not make a sale.

I was having to concentrate far harder on my driving than I used to, especially at night. Now, in the teeming rain, visibility was bad and the street lights threw distorting reflections on the road surface.

There was a fair amount of traffic about, considering the time. I stopped at a set of lights as a car slowly crossed in front of me. I watched the hunched manner and tense expression of the driver as he peered through the windscreen. He was having as much trouble with the conditions as I.

I sighed when the lights finally changed to green. I was almost home and began to relax.

I approached the last roundabout on my route – a roundabout I had negotiated so many times before.

I became confused as I neared it.

'Do you give way to the traffic waiting to join the roundabout from your left, or the traffic already on it coming from your right?' I wondered in sudden panic.

I averaged 40 000 miles a year, had spent several years as an examiner for the motorcyle proficiency test, and suddenly could not remember the priority at roundabouts. It became too late even as I pondered.

A van already on the roundabout hit me as I pulled out in front of it and wrote off my three-week-old car.

Fortunately, there were no injuries.

It was entirely my fault. I had arrived at the false conclusion that you gave way to the traffic from the left instead of the right.

Sylvia arranged an appointment with the doctor, and at last, reluctantly, I went to see him.

* * *

The waiting room was almost full when Sylvia and I arrived the following morning, and it seemed an age before the receptionist called my name. I wondered if any of the other patients suspected that I was there due to a mental problem. I kept blowing my nose loudly and rubbing my eyes, hoping that they would think I was there with a touch of flu. The middle-aged lady next to me got up and sat on another chair across the room, so perhaps my idea was working.

'Now what seems to be the problem?' Dr Ness asked when we finally went to see him.

I have always liked Dr Ness. He is the sole doctor in the practice and seems to really care about his patient's health.

We transferred here from a larger and more impersonal surgery, where you were lucky to see the same doctor on two consecutive visits. They called out your number rather than your name when the doctor, or should I say administrator, was ready to see you. 'Now what seems to be the problem?' Dr Ness repeated. I wondered if that was a standard opening remark. I tried to estimate how many times he would say that during the day in his crowded surgery.

'I said, Now what seems to be the problem?, Mr Blank'.

I wondered why he was shouting. Did he think I was deaf or something?

'Is it his hearing?' he asked Sylvia. It was then that I realised that it would have been better to answer his question instead of remaining silent playing guessing games.

'No, his hearing's all right. It's just that he seems to keep going off in a world of his own.'

She dug me in the ribs. 'Here,' she said to the doctor, 'I'll get him to answer you himself.'

'It's OK, give me time,' I said. 'I think it's my memory, doctor. A couple of weeks ago, I didn't even recognise my own daughter.'

He gave me such a thorough examination that I became concerned about all the other people waiting to see him.

Eventually, he turned to Sylvia.

'How long have you noticed this change in him?'

'I don't really know, it came on so gradually – several months at least – perhaps a year or two.'

'Hmm, and have you any idea what is wrong with him?'

'No, I was hoping you could tell me.'

'Well, I may be wrong, and it will need several tests to eliminate other causes . . .' He paused and Sylvia sat waiting patiently. I wished he would get on with it so that we could go home.

'I think', he continued at last, 'that he may have pre-senile dementia. I'd like him to see a specialist.'

'But he's only 55; that's a bit young isn't it?'

'No, pre-senile dementia can strike at any age. It IS more prevalent in the elderly, and then it's more commonly known as Alzheimer's disease. They are two names for the same condition. There have been recorded cases of Alzheimer's disease as young as 25.

'However, it's very difficult to diagnose and I am by no means certain that he has it. That is why I want a second opinion.' He looked at me as if to see if I understood what they were talking about. Did he think that I was a child or something? Nobody spoke for a moment, and then Dr Ness glanced expectantly at me as if waiting for a comment.

'OK doc. You're the boss,' I said in a terrible imitation of Bugs Bunny. I knew what Alzheimer's disease was, having seen the effect it had had on my mother just before she died. However, I wanted to make light of it and not dwell on anything until we knew what the problem was for certain.

Before we left the surgery, Dr Ness telephoned a specialist who made an appointment for me to call the following Wednesday. He suggested that Sylvia should go with me. We saw the specialist, Dr Sherpa, at Birch Hill Hospital. On our arrival, the staff were very courteous and pleasant. I felt a little uneasy. Were they so pleasant because it was a psychiatric unit and they did not want to upset anyone? Perhaps everybody who calls on a Wednesday morning has Alzheimer's disease.

I looked round the waiting room at the haggard expression of the other patients and wondered if I had begun to look like that. I picked up a magazine, but before I had had a chance to look at it, the receptionist came over to usher us into the surgery.

Dr Sherpa seemed to be very young to hold such a

responsible position, but his patient and reassuring manner seemed to have a calming effect. He prompted Sylvia with questions and listened to everything that she told him. Things that I was not aware of until then. I felt a bit embarrassed and nudged her to shut her up, but once started, everything came out in a torrent.

After an exhaustive examination, he pronounced: 'Yes, I think that you probably do have Alzheimer's disease.'

He would not know for certain until the laboratory made one or two other tests on a blood sample he had taken. However, he advised us not to pin our hopes on that because he thought that it would merely confirm his present opinion.

He started counselling us, but his words were meaningless to me. I had spent the last few days in the library researching the disease; and now to have the diagnosis confirmed left me devastated. I clutched the doctor's desk as I felt the room spinning, and went off into the dream world I had been inhabiting more and more of late.

I could hear Dr Sherpa and Sylvia talking, and understood what they were saying, but it did not seem to have any relevance to me. When they asked me questions, I waited for someone else to answer.

It was only when Sylvia poked me violently in the ribs that I snapped out of it. 'The doctor says he will give you some tablets. He wants to send your blood sample off for analysis, so will you come back to see him next week?'

I think I may have forgotten or at least ignored his previous remarks as I answered, 'Yes, I suppose so. You mean we'll get the results of the test then? Perhaps I haven't got it after all?'

Dr Sherpa looked serious and sad. He seemed concerned and it did not look like an act. 'No, as I said, I don't want you to get any false hopes up. The blood test is only a formality. I'm afraid to say that I am of the opinion that there is no doubt at all that you do have Alzheimer's disease.'

Formality or not, I was not giving up so easily. 'I thought that the only way to diagnose Alzheimer's was to dissect the brain. There is no certain way to prove that a living person has it, is there?'

'No, you're quite correct. There isn't. However, having eliminated all the other possibilities, that is the only remaining one that fits your symptoms. As the only way to diagnose it is to eliminate all other possibilities, and we have virtually done so apart from the blood test, I am afraid that that is what we are now left with.'

I muttered something and made for the door. I wanted to get out of there.

I was certain that I did not have the disease, and when my blood sample came back, the good doctor would have to agree.

I wanted to get home and not think about it any more. There really was no point in worrying about it when I was sure that we would find out it was all a mistake in a few days.

I kept my face averted so as not to catch anyone's eyes as we walked out through the reception area. There were several more people waiting there than when we arrived, and I wondered how many of them were going to receive similar news to mine. As we left through the large double doors, I glanced back briefly, and a phrase came into my mind: 'Abandon hope, all ye who enter here'. I half-expected to see it chiselled into the lintel above the door.

It was not.

When we left the hospital grounds, Sylvia took my arm to guide me across the road.

A few weeks ago, I would have taken hers.

CHAPTER THREE

Diagnosis Confirmed

✳

The following week we returned to see Dr Sherpa. I was impatient to know if he had any news. My impatience increased when, after asking me how I was, he made small talk for a few minutes before he at last got to the point.

'The analysis of your blood sample came back yesterday.' He paused and shuffled some papers on his desk. I wanted to shout for him to continue, but there was a constriction in my chest and my mouth was so dry that it was difficult to speak. I thought I might be going to have a heart attack and remember thinking that if I did, a doctor's surgery was probably the best place to have one. Eventually he continued, ' I have also received the results of your brain scan. I'm afraid that in both cases they were negative.'

'Negative! You mean I don't have Alzheimer's?'

'No, I'm sorry to say, negative meaning that you do. Remember, we were trying to eliminate all other possibilities. If the blood had shown a positive indication that there was another medical condition for your problem, then perhaps we could do something about it. As it is, there is no doubt that you have Alzheimer's disease . . .'

He would have gone on but I interrupted. 'How long then. How long have I got?'

'Well, that depends on what you mean. You could live for many years . . .'

'I'm not interested in that Dr Sherpa, what's the prognosis?' I thought that if I seemed to be dispassionate and kept it on the level of a medical discussion, he might answer my questions without any soothing waffle. 'How long do you estimate that I will retain the major portion of my mental faculties?'

'Who can say?' he began.

'You can!' I thought, 'I don't want any flannel, you're the bloody doctor, you can say!' I realised that I was being totally unfair, but wanted to lose my temper with someone. Perhaps he read my thoughts from my expression. He looked at me then continued. 'We know so little about progressive dementia. The timescale varies enormously between individuals. Some people degenerate within a matter of months, while others can go on for years. Sometimes many years.'

He paused again and looked at us both. Sylvia had said very little during the interview, leaving most of the questions to me. I asked the one question to which I already knew the answer. Perhaps I imagined that Dr Sherpa would give me a different reply from the one I dreaded.

'And does anyone ever stay the same, or even recover?'

'No, I'm afraid not. It is always a progressive degeneration. It is only the time interval that varies.'

It must be almost 50 years since I felt the way I did then. As a child, I had ridden on the big dipper at Blackpool. It was a rare treat when our junior school took a party of us out for a day at the seaside. The celebrations of VE Day were still vivid, and with Japan about to fall, it seemed that the war was finally ending. At last, the gloom of recent years showed a faint chink of light.

I was laughing and joking with the rest as the chain pulled the car up the long climb. When we neared the top and the car slowed almost to a stop, as if gathering its breath, I stood slightly to point out a landmark.

I could see the whole of the town and coast spread out below me.

The car then crested the rise, the nose dipped . . . and the world fell away from under me as the car rushed in headlong flight towards the ground so far below.

I now gripped the arms of the surgery chair as I felt the same sensation.

I remember thinking that there was one difference.

On the dipper, the mad plunge into the abyss caused screaming from all the passengers, not least myself. Now, the screams were all within my head.

I might have broken down, but one thing saved me. I heard Sylvia ask, 'And is there no cure? Can't you do anything?'

And the doctor's reply, 'No, nothing. Nothing can be done at all, there is no cure.'

That answer was my salvation.

All my life people have been telling me that I cannot do something, or that such and such a thing was impossible.

All my life I have devoted my time and energy to proving them wrong.

I spent several weeks learning all I could about Alzheimer's disease, first at my local library in Rochdale, and later at Manchester Central Library.

All the books made depressing reading, but it soon became clear that there were wide gaps in the research. While most of the authors agreed that the disease caused minute plaques to form on the surface of the brain, no one seemed to know the reason. Neurofibrillary tangles seem to be the root cause of the loss of memory. I made a note to look into this further.

The main theory seemed to link it to aluminium poisoning, but several works disagreed with this.

However, to be on the safe side, I asked Sylvia to throw out all our aluminium saucepans and we replaced them with an enamelled set.

I studied the list of contents on the items in our medicine cupboard, and put them all back except one, a bottle of Aludrox. The name alone should have given me a clue to its ingredients. As mentioned earlier, I had suffered from heartburn over the years and had taken this Aludrox, an antacid remedy, to relieve it. This was the first time I noticed that the main ingredient was aluminium hydroxide. With medical research still undecided as to whether aluminium could be a cause of Alzheimer's disease, I did not want a medicine containing it in the house. I asked Dr Ness to suggest a replacement for it, and he gave me a prescription for a similar medicine called Gaviscon that did not contain aluminium.

Further reading again implicated aluminium with the disease. I could not overlook the coincidence that aluminium was first commercially produced in its refined form in 1896, and Alois Alzheimer discovered Alzheimer's disease in 1906.

In his book, *Reducing the Risk of Alzheimer's,* Dr Michael A. Weiner stresses this link, and refers to autopsies on the brains of people who have died from the disease. These all show high concentrations of aluminium in the neurofibrillary tangles and cells in the brain tissue. Apparently, a membrane called the blood–brain barrier protects the brain from toxins, but if this barrier is ruptured, perhaps by a blow to the head, it may allow aluminium to pass into the brain. This is a slow process that may take many years to develop.

I thought back to a motorcycle accident in 1978, and wondered if it could be implicated.

Motorcycles have always been a passion with me. Over the years, I have ridden or owned many of them. I used to take part in club and vintage races and occasionally rode in club events with Chas Mortimer in the racing school he ran at Mallory Park.

Sylvia, too, has always been wildly enthusiastic about motorcycles, and as our standard of living improved, so did the quality of my bikes. We used to ride them whenever we could, and the few minor accidents we had did not put us off.

However, I suppose the head injury I received in one of the accidents may have had a part to play in my later illness.

In 1978, I was riding a V. Twin Italian bike, a metallic green Ducati 900 GTS. It had the usual atrocious Italian electrical equipment and the fixed footrests were so low that they were a constant aggravation. You just could not lean the bike far enough over to exploit its fantastic handling before they grounded.

If you did attempt to force the bike further over when this happened, the bike would pivot on the footrest, lift the rear wheel, and throw you into the ditch.

I can vouch for this.

The Italians designed it as a touring bike, and a touring bike it remained, even though the frame was so similar to the one on the machine on which Mike Hailwood won the TT. This bike had so many idiosyncrasies that every journey was an adventure that kept me wondering if I would reach my destination.

I loved that bike with a deep and burning passion.

I was riding the Ducati behind my son, Michael, who was on a Honda. Michael had just passed a line of parked vehicles when one of them, a taxicab, began pulling out of the line. Assuming that the taxi would just pull out and drive forward, I swerved to the right to pass it. However, the cabby started to do a U-turn in the road, as the reason he had pulled out was that he had seen a potential fare on the opposite pavement.

With the taxi now sideways in front of me, I swerved to the left, hoping to squeeze behind him. However, as my headlamp lit up the inside of his cab, he suddenly realised I was there, slammed on his brakes, and stopped square on in front of me.

I rarely swear, but Sylvia, who was riding pillion, says that I did so on this occasion. Hearing me over our intercom, she leapt off the back of the bike, while I smashed into the taxi and somersaulted over the bonnet.

I picked myself up on the far side of the taxi, and ran back round it to see if Sylvia was all right. (This amazed the ambulance men when they turned up as, among other injuries, I had a broken ankle.)

Fortunately, Sylvia was not hurt apart from a little bruising – which caused an inordinate amount of groaning – but as well as my ankle, I had a Colles' fracture of my wrist and a large bump on my head. This bump was not enough to cause concussion. The hospital thought it so insignificant that they did not bother to do an X-ray, and doubtless nothing would have appeared abnormal if they had. I had no other head examination until the brain scan in October 1992 that proved negative. However, as I mentioned, my later research led me to wonder if the blood–brain barrier membrane could have been damaged in this accident.

I spent a couple of weeks in hospital and my beautiful Ducati was a write-off.

I seemed to have escaped lightly, and Sylvia only had slight bruising, yet this accident hurt me deeply. It was not our injuries that bothered me – after all, I have been riding motorcycles for nearly 40 years, and have had numerous accidents on them. I rode one as a dispatch rider in the army, over such atrocious terrain that I spent more time picking the bike up than I did in the saddle. I once rode slightly faster than usual and clean over a 20-foot cliff when an unknown terrorist fired on me in Kenya; yet none of these experiences equalled the trauma this accident caused me.

After I hobbled back to ensure that Sylvia was all right, my ankle gave way and I sat down heavily.

I sat on the edge of the pavement to wait for the ambulance and looked at my Ducati. Her name was 'Boa', after 'Boanerges', the Brough Superior that Lawrence of Arabia rode and described so vividly after he raced a monoplane on her.

I swear my 'Boa' was of a similar mould. It started out as a 900 cc V. Twin, but I bored it out to 1100 cc. This was to increase the torque rather than the top end power and it achieved this admirably. I managed to raise the gear ratio to such an extent that it would rumble along happily in top gear with the engine throbbing contentedly in time with the passing lamp-posts.

Unlike so many modern bikes, Boa had a soul. And I loved her.

Now she lay broken in a pool of oil, her frame twisted and her forks bent agonisingly back into her engine.

As I watched, a red tear oozed from her brake fluid reservoir and wept gently down her headlamp casing. Even with my helmet on, I could hear the heartfelt bleats of her alarm. This was in a slim box fitted to her frame. A spectator put a stop to her howls by kicking the box violently until the noise subsided. At this point, a wisp of vapour rose from her cracked cylinder case. I dare say some of the watchers thought that it was oil vapour.

I knew it was her departing soul ascending to a motorcycle heaven.

A woman, perhaps seeing my distress, said soothingly, 'Never mind, love, you'll be able to get another bike with the insurance.'

I did not answer.

I remember once hearing a nurse in hospital telling a distraught mother who had lost her daughter to leukaemia. 'Never mind, dear, you're young enough to have another.'

A sequel to this is that, over a year later, Sylvia phoned an appliance repair company because our fridge was not working. When the man called to fix it, Sylvia thought she recognised him, but could not be sure. She went into the kitchen where he was working and offered to make a him a cup of tea. While the water was boiling, she remembered where she had seen him before. She reported the following conversation to me later.

'Didn't you used to drive a taxi?' she asked him.

'Yes, love, you've got a good memory. Did I give you a lift somewhere?'

'No, you didn't. I'll tell you what you did do though. You smashed up my husband's motorbike in an accident.'

'Oh, when was that then?'

'For God's sake, how many motorbikes have you had accidents with?'

'Oh, was yours a green un?'

'Yes, it was a "green un". It was a Ducati and I was on the back.'

'Sorry, love. By the way, you need a new evaporator for this fridge. This one's knackered.'

After he left, Sylvia told me that she had not given him any biscuits with his tea. Vindictive, huh?

Sylvia thinks it was three or four years after this that she first noticed that I was a little absent-minded. As time passed, I steadily became more forgetful, culminating with not recognising Ruth in the lift.

I now broadened my studies to take in other aspects of the brain, and it surprised me to find how little of it we use. I was aware that the brain has a far greater capacity than we use, but I had not realised how little of it we need to exist.

I became absorbed in the case of a girl who died in her late teens. She had appeared perfectly normal all her life, but at the age of 12 had had a routine X-ray of her head following a fall. The medical staff at the hospital could not believe what it showed at first, so they ordered another one.

This confirmed that she had no brain as such at all. A fatty deposit and liquid appeared to fill her cranium instead of a normal brain.

They gave her numerous tests and proved her to be literate, numerate and of average intelligence. On her death, a post-mortem confirmed that she did not have a brain, just a thickening of the brain stem.

I found this fascinating and concluded that a person with half, or even a quarter, of a normally functioning brain should do at least as well as she. I carried on with my studies with renewed determination. It amazed me how much conflicting evidence there was in the medical books. I read several that stated that plaques and neurofibrillary tangles were conclusive evidence of Alzheimer's disease; then, in another book, I read that even normal brains exhibit these symptoms with ageing, though not to the same degree. However, it suggested to me that the diagnosis of the disease during a post-mortem was more of a subjective judgement than I had thought.

My research took me down many blind alleys and I read about many claims that appeared bogus. These ranged from the false benefits of massive doses of megavitamins to obscure herbal remedies. Some of them looked promising until I studied them in more detail.

I wondered whether a restricted flow of blood to the brain might be a contributory factor in the disease. I therefore studied the results of vasodilators that the medical profession occasionally uses to increase the blood flow. However, these seem to do more harm than good. They work by dilating the blood vessels, thus allowing the blood to flow more freely. However, as they also dilate peripheral blood vessels in the limbs, they can reduce rather than increase the flow to the brain.

I made a note to check whether vasodilators would help if used in conjunction with transfusions of additional blood. If this seemed likely, I foresaw a dilemma ahead. There had been several newspaper articles about people contracting AIDS through contaminated blood. I would not want to risk blood transfusions that might help with one problem and then cause another.

My main dilemma now seemed to be a short attention span. I found it difficult to concentrate for extended periods. There was also a problem with my awareness of time. I would take some books out of the library and a day or two later, before I had a chance to look at them properly, Sylvia would ask me if I wanted them renewed as they were due back. I took a lot of convincing that three weeks had gone by without my knowledge. On other days, I found a week's growth of beard on my chin, when I was certain that I had shaved that very morning.

One day, I left the house intending to see if our local W.H. Smith's had any relevant books. The shortest route is through the local market, which was at its busiest peak when I arrived, with milling and jostling people scrambling to get to the stalls.

It was merely drizzling when I entered the indoor market, which was unusually gloomy as the faint daylight fought its way through the translucent plastic roof.

In spite of the weather, the market was full of people mooching about in search of a bargain.

Suddenly, it became glaringly bright as a streak of lightning hit the building and sizzled along one of the aluminium channels separating the plastic sheets on the roof. The plastic warped slightly and rain started to pour through a gap. There came a crack of thunder, and everybody cowered as they thought that the roof was going to collapse in on them. In panic, everyone struggled and fought their way to the exits. The crowd hemmed me in on all sides and carried me along.

The screaming bedlam seemed to press in on me. The throng hemmed me in, and everyone seemed to be shouting at once. The wave of noise overwhelmed me and I stopped as the crowd trapped me against a supporting pillar. I stood there with my hands over my ears. I could not think or move and shouted out, '**BE QUIET! SHUT UP! LET'S HAVE A BIT OF PEACE AND QUIET, FOR GOD'S SAKE.**'

The people rushing by were looking at me, and I realised how ridiculous my shouting was, but could not help myself.

Then my legs came back to life and I ran.

I ran, pushing and shoving my way out of the pandemonium in the market.

I may have knocked one or two people over; I neither knew nor cared. I did not know I was capable of it, but I ran all the way home. Fortunately, the door was on the latch. If it had been locked, I think I would have put my shoulder to it, rather than fumble with a key. I ran in the house and into my den where I sank down to regain my breath. I did not venture out of the house for two weeks, and then I had to return after a few tentative steps.

I got worse and developed full-blown agoraphobia and could not leave the house at all. I could no longer bear to be in the hall if the front door was open. At its peak, I found even our small sitting room was too large for comfort and spent most of the time in my tiny den.

However, my major problem was with my memory. I seemed to be getting so forgetful, even with things that had just happened. I sometimes went into a room for something and stood there wondering what I came in to get.

This was not just the occasional momentary lapse that everyone has from time to time; it happened so frequently. Take one day, for instance. I had been up most of the night, and had gone to bed at about half past five in the morning. Sylvia was already up when I awoke. I got out of bed and began to get dressed, sitting on the bed to put on my socks.

I must have started daydreaming or something because I came to with a start and could not remember whether I was getting up or going to bed. It was still dark out so I thought it must be night time, put my pyjamas on and got back into bed.

A few minutes later Sylvia came in to tell me that breakfast was ready, so I had to get dressed twice in one day. The strange thing is, I really felt as though she had got me up just after I went to bed, and I still felt tired.

*   *   *

A few weeks after seeing Dr Sherpa, another doctor came to examine me. The examination had to be at home because my agoraphobia had worsened. He introduced himself as Dr Moorland. After asking Sylvia many questions, he eventually turned to me. Determined to prove that I was not ill, I tried to look as attentive and intelligent as possible.

After asking a few preliminary questions such as my name and age, etc., Dr Moorland asked me the name of the prime minister. 'Margaret Thatcher', I replied promptly.

'And what day is it?'

'Tuesday'.

'Good, now I want you to subtract seven from 100, then subtract seven from that and so on.'

This was so childishly easy. He just wanted me to count down from 100 in sevens. I had always been good at maths, why could he not give me something a bit more difficult as a test?

'Well, go on then,' he said.

I realised that I had been musing instead of answering his question. This would never do. I must try to answer his questions promptly. As a schoolchild, I had always tried to put my hand up first when the teacher asked the class a question. I remember one day at school when . . .

Dr Moorland interrupted my train of thought. 'Have you worked out the answer?' he asked.

'Yes, of course!' I said. 'Now what was it you wanted to know?'

'I want you to take seven away from 100. Just do it the once to begin with.'

'Right then. 100 minus seven is . . . Er, is . . .' I could not do it! It was as though simple arithmetic was a strange language that I had never learned. The more I strained, the harder it got. I wiped my forehead and tried again. He was talking to me but I could not pause to understand what he was trying to say. I had to solve this simple problem. He put his hand on my arm and repeated himself. This time I relaxed and listened to him.

'Don't treat it as a sum, look at it this way. If I had £100 and gave you seven, what would I have left?'

I still could not work it out, and listened to myself in horror as I tried to distract him. I was talking like a stupid child. 'I don't know what you'd have left, but if you had £100 and gave me seven, I'd go out and buy some sweets.'

He did not reply, but just put away his notepad and rose to leave.

Sylvia went to see him out and I could hear their conversation in the hall. 'Well, that confirms it, I'm afraid.'

'Are you sure? I mean, this is just one of his bad days. Sometimes he is much better than this.'

'I am afraid there is very little room for doubt,' he said as I heard him opening the front door. 'He didn't even know the name of the prime minister.'

Sylvia seemed to lose her temper. I heard her shouting after him. 'If forgetting John Major's name is regarded as proof of illness, then we'll all be hospitalised within ten years.'

She was crying when she returned. 'Stupid doctor. What does he know?'

'I didn't do too bad, did I?' I asked.

'You couldn't have done much worse, darling. You didn't get one question right.'

'What questions did I get wrong then?'

'All of them. You told him it's Tuesday, and it's Thursday. Then when he asked you how old you are, you said 34. Ruth's older than that.'

'Who's Ruth?'

She would not answer me but just burst out sobbing.

CHAPTER FOUR

Agoraphobia

*

Sylvia and I often used to go shopping together but, unfortunately, she now has to go alone.

One day, she came home distraught.

She was on the way to the shops when a youth, aged about 14 or so, cycled past her and snatched her hand-bag.

He rode off out of sight, and although two men gave chase, they could not catch him. She went to the police station to report it, but they were not very helpful.

She said that she had to wait ages before she could speak to anyone, and then the constable at the desk just wrote it in the incident book as a formality. One of the other policemen told her that he doubted whether they would catch the thief, but even if they did, there was nothing they could do to him other than give him a cau-tion. He said that the last time his inspector had cautioned a young boy, the lad just stuck his tongue out at him and walked off as if he owned the place.

Sylvia says that she does not know how we will manage this week because she had our week's pension in her bag, but I know we will get through somehow; we always do. It still worries me though, and not just because we lost a bit of money. This time it was a young lad who robbed her, but it could easily have been an older youth or an adult, who might have mugged her or worse.

I feel so bad about it that I do not want to let Sylvia go shopping alone; but I cannot go with her. I start to shake as soon as I leave the house, and I am sure that if I walked a few steps away, I would pass out.

I was miserable for the rest of the day, and went to bed early hoping that I would feel better when I woke up.

* * *

Early the next morning, I awoke in terror.

Covered in sweat yet shivering with cold, I would have thought that I had malaria if I had been back in Africa.

I was in a state of pure panic.

I had pushed the thought of Alzheimer's disease to the back of my mind during the day, but now the full implications came home to me. The thought of losing my memory and my ability to reason horrified me.

Not being of even average ability at physical sports had never really bothered me. So what if I was not a world-class athlete. It was my mind I was proud of, and now I was about to lose it. It would be even worse for Sylvia.

I would eventually not even realise I was ill, but I would be an increasing burden to her.

As I lay there in bed waiting for the first glimmer of dawn, dark thoughts of the future bore down on me. I clutched the mattress through the sheet as the room began to spin, and lay there stiff with panic until Sylvia must have sensed my distress and came in to comfort me.

After breakfast, I stood on the balcony of our flat and looked out over the town. I felt at peace on the balcony, with no trace of agoraphobia. My thoughts returned to the depressing prospect I had dwelt on earlier.

Most suffers of Alzheimer's disease are relatively happy because, in the early stages, there is a form of self-delusion and they do not admit to themselves they they have it. However, in the later stages, their mind itself can no longer appreciate the enormity of their illness.

It is the person caring for the victim who suffers most, as they gradually see a loved one slip away from them. I did not want Sylvia to work and slave to look after me for 24 hours a day, all the while knowing that eventually I would not even recognise her, or realise that she was my wife. It was something that I could not put her through. The disease could take several years to run its course, and Sylvia deserved better than to have the latter part of her life ruined by me.

I put both my hands on the balcony rail and looked at the Pennine hills in the distance.

They were just a faint smudge on the horizon that formed a natural boundary between my home of Lancashire and neighbouring Yorkshire.

The Battle of the Roses has long been forgotten, but there is still a jocular rivalry between the two counties. 'To give it its due, Yorkshire is a wonderful county,' regulars at the local pub would announce loudly if they heard a Yorkshire accent in the bar, 'we won't hear a word said against it. It keeps all the wind off Lancashire.'

I looked down at the ground so far below. The whole of Rochdale lay spread out below me. In the distance I could see the cars crawling along the M62 motorway, and beyond that the dark smudge that was the northern edge of Manchester. Below me, I could see the tiny dots of people hurrying to and from the market. Just across the road was the cricket pitch with a match in progress.

I often used to watch the cricket through binoculars, but sadly that will soon be a thing of the past. A large supermarket chain bought the land and intend to turn it into yet another supermarket. We already have more than our fair share of them and it sickens me the way some people put commerce before so many of the better things of life. Not that I am an avid cricket fan, far from it. It is just one of so many examples of how the life of local communities is deteriorating.

The cricket field provides quiet enjoyment to so many people.

So many things are changing these days . . . so few for the better.

I watched a couple of seagulls as they wheeled and dived before me. 'Must be a storm at sea,' I muttered, aware that seaguls normally only flew this far inland to escape bad weather. They swooped down towards the tower block on which I stood, then hovered in front of me in the updraught of air.

The wind was mild on my face, and as I held my hand over the balcony, I could distinctly feel the warm updraught between my fingers. I waved my hand in imitation of their flight as I thought about the problem that had been bothering me lately.

I was becoming more and more of a burden to Sylvia, and that was nothing to the grief I would cause her in the later stages of my illness. Sylvia had enough troubles of her own; she was a diabetic and had chronic arthritis.

I sighed and wondered how she would possibly cope.

I could faintly hear the sound of applause carried up on the wind and guessed that a fielder had probably made a spectacular catch on the cricket field below. One player would be feeling very proud while the other would be miserable. C'est la vie!

I leaned over the balcony and looked down to see if I could make out what had occurred on the playing field and was surprised at the strength of the updraught.

It ruffled my hair and felt like a physical force. No wonder the birds could soar on it so easily. 'Why,' I thought, 'I bet it could even support me.'

I watched the nearest gull diving and soaring, and to my mind it took on the appearance of an eagle. An eagle I had seen many years before. Suddenly, I was no longer standing on the balcony of a tower block in Rochdale.

In my mind, I was transported back to the time when I was a much younger man in Kenya, standing looking out over the Rift Valley.

Although almost 40 years had passed since I viewed the scene from a lost age when game was still plentiful in Africa, it remained etched in my memory.

I relived it in my mind.

The cliff fell vertically for just over a mile at this point, but the ground at its base sloped gently away to the valley floor and teemed with life. An eagle flew overhead and then dived to its eyrie below me in the cliff face. I watched for a while, but when it failed to reappear, I transferred my gaze to the land below. Even without binoculars, I could make out herds of golden brown impala and groups of yellow eland with their short stubby horns. I could identify the purplish brown waterbuck by the white circles on their rumps, and the tiny klipspringer darting and dancing among the larger gazelles.

The light warm African breeze now wafted up to me the fragrance of mimosa and jasmine. Even these heady perfumes could not overcome the hot dusty smell of the red earth of the African savannah. The air was clear and so fresh that my nostrils tingled as I breathed it in deeply. Every varied scent of the morning was distinct. The heavy fragrance of the solanum blooms contrasted sharply with the damp woody smell of the tree against which I leaned. Its bole had long ago been cloven in two by a lightning strike, yet still it survived almost as two separate trunks. The rough bark pressed against my back and I felt a deep empathy with the sylvan spirit within the tree.

About a couple of miles away, there was a stand of huge podocarpus trees. I recalled how surprised I was to learn that these mountains of living wood were cousins of the far smaller cedar trees they had in England. Nearer at hand, lava boulders and 'wait-a-bit' thorn bushes covered the ground. Between them stood a Cape chestnut tree covered with a mass of cyclamen-pink panicles.

The only sounds were the faint sighing of the breeze, and the ever-present chirruping of the cicada beetles.

There were so many wonderful things in the world, why did there have to be such sorrow as well?

A car sounded its horn far below me, and I was back in Rochdale. My eyesight seemed to have sharpened, and I could make out another player coming in to bat.

The cricket pitch, 400 yards or so across the road, was about twice the distance away from my tower block as my height was above the ground. About a 45-degree angle, I guessed.

Fairly steep for a car to climb, but a gentle glide for a bird. Why, with this strong updraught, I bet I could almost glide down there myself. Now that would be something. I imagined the astonished faces of the players and spectators as I glided gently down on to the pitch in front of them. The umpire would not like it. I could visualise his stern expression as he raised his finger to signal a foul.

'No, wait a minute,' I thought as I climbed higher on the balcony railing to see better, 'they don't have fouls in cricket. That's football.' I could not imagine what they had in cricket. 'That's not cricket!' I could imagine him saying.

I lifted my arms to imitate the nearby seagull. he was floating effortlessly only a few feet in front of me, and I was sure he was watching me. He wa so close I could see his staring eye, and I stared back into it as I gently flapped my arms . . . then fell backwards as Sylvia yanked my collar.

I banged my head on the ground and shouted out, 'What did you do that for?' She did not say anything but pushed me indoors. She seemed furious with me. I was the one who should be annoyed. She should not have dragged me back in like that.

It was so peaceful out there.

I have tried to go out on the balcony several times since, but the door is always locked and Sylvia says that she has lost the key. I think I could get it open if I could find my tool box but that has gone as well.

Sylvia is always losing things these days. She really should be more careful.

✻   ✻   ✻

My agoraphobia has eased lately, and Sylvia and I are now able to go out for short walks together. It makes such a pleasant change from being cooped up indoors. We still avoid the market when it is busy, and other crowded places, just to be on the safe side.

Yesterday, we met Colin while we were out shopping. He used to be the caretaker in our block of flats, but his doctor rushed him into hospital a few months ago for major surgery. Many of us doubted whether we would ever see him again, but fortunately he pulled through and is now fully recovered. He looks entirely different though, so thin and drawn. He seems to have given up smoking which many of us felt was a cause of his problem.

He had changed so much that when he spoke to us, Sylvia did not recognise him at first. Neither did I, but at least she now knows what it feels like not to know the identity of a person who is talking to you.

I have not written anything for a couple of days as I have been trying to sort out a problem with my computer.

All things electronic, especially computers, fascinate me. I like discovering how they work, and adapting them for my needs in ways the manufacturer did not intend. After I wrote a number of programs in BASIC and games in C+, I found debugging computers very enthralling, especially after I built up my first real computer, an 8086, to its present configuration of a 486Dx2.

Early this week, I turned it on and it failed to start up properly. It took me two days to discover the reason. I had temporarily altered my 'Config.Sys' file to create a virtual disk, and before doing so had renamed the 'Config.Sys' as 'Config.Old'. It took me two days to realise that when I renamed it back, I had spelled 'Config' as 'Conffig'. At one time this would have taken me two minutes, or more probably I would not have misspelled it in the first place.

* * *

My illness seemed to be fluctuating, but gradually gettng worse. Occasionally, I became quite lucid and like my normal self. At other times, I deteriorated until I was almost illiterate and innumerate. My moods also varied. Sometimes I was happy; deliriously happy and laughed and sang for no reason. At other times, I was in a deep depression and sat in silence.

For several weeks, I had been keeping a diary, but now found that several pages were blank. I also became aware of difficulties with typing and speling, and had to consult a dictionary over quite simple words.

I ocazionally became vilently angry, feeling that i had somehow had a portion of my life stolen from me.

My typing slowed dramatically, and i found it more difficult to use ht dictionary as i didn't no how too look ht wods up. slyvia notised this and has agred to crect my speling and gramer from now on.

* * *

Sylvia became worried about us living on the eleventh floor of a tower block. I think the height really bothered her and that is why she kept the balcony door locked. One day, she went to the council offices to see whether they could move us to a ground-floor flat. There were none vacant, but she filled in a card for their files and the lady told us that they would notify us if one became available. Sylvia also mentioned to our doctor that she did not like living in a high-rise flat.

We thought nothing more of it until, several months later, we received a printed postcard asking us if we still wanted them to keep us on the register of property exchanges. Sylvia ticked the box marked 'Yes' and returned it.

The following week, the phone rang. It was the housing office telling us that they had a bungalow that was vacant, and we could pick up the keys if we wanted to view it. My agoraphobia had been getting better lately, and the chance of moving to a bungalow excited us so much that I did not hesitate when she asked me if I wanted to go with her.

We picked up the keys and went to have a look at it.

We walked from the council offices as the new address was not far, and passed several council bungalows on the way. They were in blocks of seven or eight, and we wondered if ours would be like one of them. 'I hope ours is on the end of a terrace,' Sylvia said. 'That way it will almost be like a semi.'

When we arrived at the road named on the card, we thought at first that we had got the address wrong. There did not seem to be any bungalows, just houses that, judging by the different doors and windows, were privately owned. We walked down the road checking the numbers, and when we saw our bungalow, Sylvia gasped.

It was an adorable little cottage, set back from the road and completely detached in its own gardens. The front garden was very small but the one at the side was a little larger. A flowering cherry tree stood by the front door.

At the rear, there was a much larger garden that was presently overgrown with flowering currant bushes and forsythia.

We fell in love with our new home immediately, even before we opened the front door.

It had just the one bedroom, a bathroom, a kitchen and a lounge. We were glad to see that there was room to fit a small dining table in the kitchen. We both prefer to sit at a table for our meals, and not eat in the modern way with a plate balanced on a knee while viewing the television.

It was a fairly new building, even though it smelt a little musty. It had been vacant for several months as the piles of papers and circulars in the hall testified.

We rushed back to the council office before they closed and said that we would take it.

This was on a Tuesday, and the council lady told us that we would have to move in on the following Monday. This suited us, but we could not understand what all the rush was for, when the place had been empty for months.

When we originally moved into the flat from our house in Shawclough we had had to sell off most of our furniture as there was no room for it. We now realised that we could not even bring what little we had left with us because our new home was so small. We did not mind. With our children now grown up, there were only the two of us and this cosy bungalow was ideal.

I measured it from the outside recently, and confirmed what I had previously thought. Apart from the height of the pitched roof, the whole building would have easily fitted into the lounge of our house at Shawclough.

I still do not know how or why we were given the opportunity of having this bungalow.

We had been on the exchange list for months while this place was vacant, and then had to move in such a rush.

We did not mind at all, but could not help being curious.

We just accepted that fate was being kind to us.

Our new home is a little more unusual than we thought. Originally, the site was the property of the parents of Julie Goodyear (Bet Lynch in 'Coronation Street'). They had a corner shop that was demolished to make room for the present bungalow.

Neither of us used to believe in the supernatural until one day, a few years after we were married, Sylvia told me that the place we were living in was haunted. This was a maisonette in Midhope Buildings, a gloomy block of flats at King's Cross in London. She did not seem upset about it, and told me that it seemed a friendly sort of ghost that just came and sat on the bed while she was combing her hair. She told me she had often felt it brushing past her in the bedroom, but it always seemed so friendly that it did not frighten her.

Of course I did not believe her, thinking that she was just imagining it. Then one day, I walked into the bedroom while she was sitting on the bed in front of the dressing table. She caught my eye in the mirror and put her finger to her lips, then pointed at the bed.

There was a deep depression in the bed beside her as though someone was sitting there. I thought that there must be a rational explanation, perhaps a mattress spring had broken or something, and went to put my hand on the bed.

Immediately the depression rose, for all the world as though an invisible man had just stood up, and I swear I felt something brush past me on its way to the door. It was such a casual thing, just like a member of the family passing me in the house. I realised what Sylvia meant when she said it was a friendly ghost. I felt no fear about it, then or since, just curiosity.

Now this little bungalow seems to have its own friendly ghost, so similar to the previous one that we wonder if it has followed us here. We occasionally hear it walking about upstairs, going into the bedroom and closing the door, then sitting on the bed. Sometimes we hear it getting up in the morning and coming downstairs.

Yes, I know this is a bungalow, but obviously our ghost does not. There may be a rational explanation, but I cannot think of one. If it is a ghost he (somehow we both think of it as a 'he') does not bother us; in fact we would rather like to meet him.

We feel very comfortable in our little bungalow, despite a few problems when we first arrived here. The first of these was with the telephone. We arranged with BT to have the phone connected the day before we moved in. On the day of the move, we went to the new house by taxi, and Sylvia left me there to let the gas man in when he called to connect the meter. She returned in the cab to wait for the removal van. She said that she would phone me every hour.

The gas man came, connected the meter, and asked to use the phone.

'The line's dead, not to worry, it isn't important,' he said as he left. I did worry. I was alone in a strange, empy house, and it terrified me. The tiny house seemed to grow and grow until it now appeared to be enormous without any furniture in it. I hid in the cloak cupboard until Sylvia arrived and found me.

BT sent us a cheque for £50 because they had not connected the line as promised.

I would not go through that again for £50 000.

Our troubles with the new house did not stop there. As I said, it's a lovely little house, but we have had more than our fair share of teething problems with it.

Sylvia shot out of bed in the middle of the first night as water burst through the ceiling and drenched her. We spent the next few hours mopping up and putting bowls under the dripping ceiling until a plumber arrived the following morning. He went into the loft, fiddled about for a bit and eventually stopped the leak.

He told us that the cause was that the house had been empty for a long time and all the joints in the central heating pipes in the loft had dried out and shrunk. He reassured us that we would have no more troubles with leaks from the loft.

Unfortunately, that was not the case. Sylvia woke up the next night saying that she could hear something dripping.

We found the cause when we squelched on the sodden carpets in the lounge. The ceiling was leaking. Again we were up all night, mopping up and emptying bowls of water until a plumber arrived. Fortunately, it was a different man, or we might never have found out the true reason. The other plumber had trodden on a water pipe in the loft and fractured it.

That still was not the end of the trouble. We had ANOTHER flood from the loft two nights later. This time it was the ball valve in the water tank that had stuck and caused the tank to overflow.

A few days after we moved in, two ladies, a social worker and a psychiatric nurse, came to see us. They had a couple of forms for Sylvia to complete.

They stayed most of the morning and asked Sylvia many questions about me.

Before they left, they gave us a cassette containing a relaxation programme, with instructions that I was to listen to it every day to prevent 'panic attacks'. It was a beautiful day and our neighbour was out polishing his car as they were leaving. He was carrying on a conversation with the widow across the road who was clipping her hedge. They stopped talking to look at our two visitors as they were leaving.

'Good-bye,' Sylvia shouted as they were getting in the car.

'Good-bye, see you again soon,' the social worker shouted back.

The psychiatric nurse called out loudly through the car window as she drove past our neighbour, 'Good-bye, and don't worry about him too much, love. None of us are completely sane.' Sylvia closed the door quickly.

* * *

One morning I had only been typing for a short while and found that I could not read what I had just written. There was not one word that made sense. I became convinced that my computer had misspelled them all on purpose and flew into a rage.

I picked up the computer and slammed it down on the floor. It does not work any more.

Sylvia has promised to write this by hand until I get it mended.
She need not have bothered. Several days passed without me giving her anything to write. Then a man came to fix my computer. He put in a new motherboard and power pack. I was very ashamed about this because at one time I would have been able to fix it myself and save the expense. Then again, I would not have accidentally dropped it in the first place.

Fortunately, the hard disk was OK, so I had not lost all my software programs.

While he was fixing it I went into the garden because I could not bear to watch someone messing about with my computer.

I had been unwell for the past week, but it was such a lovely sunny day that I began to feel better and my throbbing headache was now all but gone.

It had rained in the night and I breathed in the clean fresh smell of the air. Soon the jasmine and lilac, that had so attracted Sylvia when she had first seen them, would be adding their scent.

The only flowers that had begun to show so far were some yellow tulips in the border under the grey stone wall.

Winter had finally gone, and the buds were just starting to open. The dew still lingered in the shadow of our silver birch, and a pair of starlings sang to each other in its branches.

Sylvia is very fond of her garden, and planted new bulbs shortly after we moved here. I did not know that she had planted any tulips and I walked over to examine them as they looked a bit odd.

The yellow tightly coiled blooms were peeking through out of their green jackets, but instead of standing straight and tall as tulips should, they were all hanging their heads in shame. They reminded me of a platoon of exhausted soldiers on parade to listen to a tirade from their sergeant-major.

I felt so sorry for them, and did not want Sylvia to see them standing as though in disgrace. I got some fine twine out of the greenhouse, and split a thin piece of bamboo into slivers. After I tied the splints round the tulip stems, I stood back to admire my work. They all stood proud and tall, as though they had just received an accolade from their commander-in-chief.

I thought that I would probably be able to remove the splints in a day or two and they would still stand upright.

Sylvia was very upset when she saw them the next day because the heads of the flowers had all dropped off.

'What have you done to them?' she shouted.

Then she began to cry. This caused me to weep as well, and I put my arms round her.

We stayed in the garden just holding and comforting each other for a long time.

She is very fond of her flowers, but I did not know that they were daffodils.

★ CHAPTER FIVE ★

Children –
and a Challenge!

※

I saw my Grandchildren today,
Merrily laughing in their play,
I was so happy, my heart was dancing,
As I watched the children prancing,
There are many sorrows on life's highways,
And rare golden moments of deep pleasure.
Countless, the pitfalls on fate's byways,
Few enough the gifts, to store and treasure.

Life, unkind in many ways,
Has its dark and dismal days,
But let fate bring on what it may;
I saw my Grandchildren today.

Ruth and Philip brought my grandchildren round to
see me this morning. It was like old times as they played
and scrambled all over me. We played hide-and-seek
and chased each other all over the house. All except
James, of course. He is 15 and much too old for that sort
of thing. Playing with the children soon exhausted me.

I used to be full of vigour and always on the go, but
these days I do not seem to have any energy. Dressing
myself in the morning seems to tire me out. I do have a
little more difficulty than most because, due to my
artificial hip, I have less mobility in one leg and have to
strain to put on my left sock and shoe. It used to be a
minor problem, but now it seems that the act of getting

up is enough to wear me out for the day and I am immediately ready to go back to bed again!

I did not realise how much they had tired me out until after they had gone and I had to lie down for a rest.

When I awoke, it cheered me to recall something I had seen on television several years ago. A one-legged athlete removed his false leg and hopped round a running track.

He then hopped up to, and jumped over, a 5-foot-high bar. It was amazing to see how well he coped with his handicap. The average two-legged man would have difficulty in competing with him. Many of nature's handicaps can be overcome, or at least negated, with thought and perseverance. I reflected how blind people compensated with their other senses. If the disease was destroying part of my brain, I would train the remainder to compensate.

First though, I would try to reverse, or at least curtail, the progress of the disease.

I have always believed in 'mind over matter' and know that many people have cured themselves of illness. If the brain can cure illnesses in its host body, then it should certainly be capable of curing itself.

I read everything I could find about neurofibrillary tangles and the plaques on the surface of the brain. If I was going to fight this thing, I had to know my enemy.

Reading about it was not enough. I now had to visualise it to understand it properly.

I hard boiled an egg and ground the shell into minute pieces that were almost a powder, yet still identifiable as separate pieces under my small home microscope. Then I mixed some Araldite and heated it so that it became liquid.

I now had to work quickly before it set. I carefully cracked a walnut and extracted the kernel, which I coated in the Araldite and then rolled in the ground eggshell.

While the glue was setting, I searched for as many varied types of string, wool, cotton and sisal as I could find. The sisal, being so coarse and hairy, seemed especially suitable. I separated its strands then mixed it with all the other wool, string and cotton.

I decided it needed still more tangling, so put it all in a bucket of water to soak, then poured the liquid off and mixed the rest thoroughly with my electric paint mixer.

I put it in the airing cupboard to dry, and went to see how the walnut was getting on.

The Araldite had almost set, but to be on the safe side, I decided to leave everything overnight and continue in the morning.

Amazingly, considering the determination I began with, I then forgot all about it for a couple of days – until Sylvia found the mess in the airing cupboard.

'Did you put all this rubbish in here?'

It came back to me. 'Yes, but it's not rubbish, don't throw it out. I want to do something with it after lunch.'

I began that afternoon, but instead of taking the hour or two that I had visualised, the string was so tangled and knotted that it kept me occupied for three days. I carefully, very carefully, teased out each separate length of wool, cotton, string and sisal. I took my time and sometimes spent several hours on a single fibre. It was not the result that was important but the pains that I took with the task.

Each time I got a piece untangled, I complimented myself and tried to feel good about it. I tied a variety of small items such as washers and bolts to one end of each small length as I separated it from the tangled mess, and taped the other end to a shelf so that it would hang down and straighten.

Eventually, when all the lengths were free and hanging from the shelf, I lifted each weight in turn to see if the string or cotton, etc. was still kinked or twisted.

Most of them were, so I put heavier weights on them and warmed them with Sylvia's hair dryer until they straightened.

When they were all without kinks, I looped the lengths over my hands and admired them, stroking them to feel their texture. It may sound crazy but I was attempting to teach my subconscious mind that straight fibres are preferable to tangled ones.

Then I turned to the walnut. This was much more difficult, but the harder it was and the more I had to concentrate, the better. With the aid of my microscope, a pair of surgical tweezers and a scalpel, I removed each tiny fragment of eggshell. It was essential that I did not scratch or cut the nut. I had to soften the glue with water and it took several more days to cut all the shell and Araldite off; but eventually the kernel was free of it all and I sat looking at it.

It looked remarkably like a brain. A healthy brain. I felt a glow of pride and encouraged the feeling. I told myself that not even a surgeon could have removed the shell and glue any better than I had. I did not stint my praise, and congratulated myself and admired the kernel for over an hour. It looked so much better without the foreign material stuck all over it.

I stored the memory of those last few days. I would probably need to recall it many times in the future.

I rose at about 5.30 a.m. the next morning. I have never needed much sleep: four hours a night was usually sufficient. I went into the kitchen to make some toast.

After cutting two slices and popping them under the grill, I still had a couple of hours to work on my problem before Sylvia got up. I opened the window and sniffed the air. It had been raining but the sky was clear and I searched the sky for Orion. I could not find it, as the constellations seemed different. They refused to take on their familiar shapes. I could not even find the plough. The stars seemed to have a random pattern, as though I was viewing them for the first time. I knew that Alzheimer's disease disorientates the sufferer, and wondered if this was a symptom of it.

There was an odour in the air I could not at first place. It smelled as though someone had a bonfire, but of course no one would have one this early. I shut the window to cut out the smell. The burning smell seemed even stronger. It had a familiar odour, but not that of a bonfire. No, come to think of it, it was not a bonfire it was . . . My God! The toast! I burnt my fingers as I grabbed the handle and doused the flaming toast in the sink.

I wiped the grill pan, cut some more bread, and popped it under the grill. I stood watching it for a while but my burnt fingers tingled so I ran them under the cold tap and then put some butter on them. I picked up the burnt toast and put it in the trash can. Even after I closed the lid, the smell of the burnt bread still lingered – and became stronger.

I took the burnt toast out of the trash can and wrapped it in cling film before putting it back. It was no use, the smell worsened, and then I realised why as flames appeared from under the grill.

I put the second lot of toast with the first and cut some more bread. I watched the toast very carefully this time to make sure it did not burn.

The kitchen stank of burnt toast, and it occurred to me that it might wake Sylvia. She might even think the house was on fire. I closed the kitchen door to stop the smell escaping, then wondered if it was already too late.

Perhaps the smell was already in the hall on the way to the bedroom.

I opened the door and went into the hall, closing the door behind me. No, I could not smell burning from out here.

But I could as soon as I went back into the kitchen.

I could also see the flames from the latest lot of toast. I was not beaten yet. There was another loaf in the bread bin. It was beginning to brown nicely when a piercing whistle disturbed my concentration.

The smoke alarm in the hall had eventually woken up and gone off with a piercing shriek.

I opened the front door and waved a newspaper under the smoke alarm to stop the noise.

By the time I had fixed it, the last lot of toast had burnt and the grill pan handle had melted.

I saw the funny side a couple of days later, but at the time, I was very despondent. I used to pride myself on my cooking, not the everyday stuff – I leave that to Sylvia – but for a special occasion I would make Tournedos Rossini, Steak Diane and suchlike.

And here I was unable to concentrate long enough to make a couple of slices of toast.

Sylvia got up to see what the commotion was and cooked me an early breakfast. I tried to explain to her what had happened, but she was tight-lipped and did not seem to want to make conversation.

*　　*　　*

For the next couple of months, I practised mental exercises for three hours every morning. For the first hour and a half, I concentrated on how I had unravelled the string, and for the second period, I recalled how I had removed the flakes of eggshell from the walnut.

When I say I concentrated, I mean just that. If anyone had seen me, they would probably have thought, by my puckered forehead and contorted face, that I was in agony. Considering it a life or death situation, I gave it everything I had and felt drained at the end of the session.

I thought I could train my brain to unravel the neurofibrillary tangles and rid itself of the plaques by recalling how great it felt when each piece of twine became unravelled, and how good the walnut looked when I had cleaned it.

I am converting this section to hidden text so that it will not show on the computer screen when Sylvia looks at it later.

When I, or more likely Sylvia, finally prints this manuscript out, it will appear as hard copy; but I do not want her to read it until then.

I have realised that I am on the wrong track. The mental exercises are having no effect at all and I am getting worse each week.

I feel waves of fog overwhelming my mind and I have to struggle to think. I have not told Sylvia, but I wonder how much longer it will be before she realises. I will continue my research and try to find another way of combating this disease, but regret having wasted so much time on a fruitless exercise.

End of hidden text.

Sylvia suggested an evening out might cheer us both up. I thought she meant a meal followed by a visit to a theatre or cinema, but she had other ideas.

She wanted to go dancing. We met each other at a dance hall in 1959, and until a few years ago, used to go dancing fairly often. Sylvia was a gold medallist in Latin American and Modern Ballroom when we met, but I soon dragged her down to my bronze standard. I enjoy a waltz, foxtrot or ballroom jive, but that's my lot.

It's becoming difficult these days to find somewhere that caters for our type of dancing. We both like a decent-size dance floor where we can really step out, but these days the management usually reserves such places for sequence dancing, which is something we do not do.

We found a dance hall advertised at the Forum Centre Wythenshawe, south Manchester that sounded just right.

It was everything that we expected – a very good band and the dancing of a high standard. However, I feel that I really let Sylvia down and embarrassed her. I just could not remember any of the intricate movements we had built up together over the years. I had to think about every step instead of flowing with the music, and eventually ended up like a real beginner doing the most basic waltz steps and muttering, 'Forward side together. Forward side together.'

I know Sylvia has a lot to put up with these days, but it's such a pity that she cannot now enjoy such a simple pleasure as dancing with me any longer.

I suggested taking private dancing lessons as we used to many years ago. She seemed doubtful at first, but I persisted and she says that she will think about it.

* * *

This morning I fell out of bed and awoke in a panic not knowing where I was.

However, this was nothing new.

Have you ever awoken at night in a strange bedroom, perhaps while on holiday in a hotel, and not been able to get your bearings?

Imagine then the feeling if every morning you awoke disorientated and could not find your way around your own home.

That was my condition now.

Sylvia resorted to putting notices on all the doors, Toilet – Kitchen – Bedroom, etc. Without them, it was a case of trying every door until I eventually hit the one I wanted.

I eventually lost my sense of direction, both in the house and outdoors, to such an extent that if I walked alone out of sight of the house by more than a few metres, I would have great difficulty in finding my way back.

We temporarily solved one of my minor problems with my memory though. Previously, when I went out for a walk with Sylvia and we met anyone, I did not join in the conversation because I could not remember who they were and did not want to make a fool of myself.

We now had a rule that she would address anybody we met by name. During the conversation, she would also ask after every member of their family by name, until she saw that it had dawned on me who they were and I could then join in.

However, this success did not last long as eventually, even despite Sylvia's promptings, I could no longer recall having known the person previously.

People's faces all seemed the same to me these days, with no distinguishing characteristics.

This is especially frustrating because a few years ago I did a bit of portrait painting and learnt to study faces in detail. Now, although I can see the features, the moment I look away, I have forgotten them.

This is true in every case. Even my next-door neighbour whom I might have seen that very morning would be a stranger to me in the afternoon. Soon I did not want to go out at all and became a bit of a recluse.

Until one day we did go out and I wished we had not.

Sylvia is a diabetic and has arthritis. I did not want to be a burden on her when I got too bad, so insisted that

she follow the doctor's advice and take me to a day centre where there was occupational therapy.

My idea was that when I became too much of a hand-
ful, she could take me there just to give her a few hours'
rest each day. This first visit was just to see what the
place was like . . . We left in a hurry.

The place stank of urine and the 'therapy' consisted
of making party hats out of paper and crayoning in exercise books. Many of the patients were sitting with vacant
faces; some with tell-tale puddles under their chairs.
They obviously sat like that all day as if they were zom-
bies. I would rather be dead than arrive at the stage
where I was scrawling with crayons or sitting in such
total boredom all day.

The next morning, feeling miserable, I noticed
Sylvia's evening bag in a drawer: a dress bag covered in
black sequins. I looked at it and tried to remember what
it reminded me of. Then I realised that it looked as I had
imagined the surface of my brain would appear with the
tiny plaques covering my brain.

I stared at the bag in fascinated horror, then took it to
my workbench to shine my bench spotlight on it. I
looked at the glittering sequins and turned the bag to
catch the light from different angles. Although the
designer obviously intended them to beautify the bag,
the sequins began to repel and sicken me.

I took a scalpel out of my drawer and cut them all off
one by one. I then picked up a pair of tweezers and
removed all traces of the cut thread that had held
them.

When no evidence of their existence remained on the
bag, I collected all the sequins and violently ground
them to a fine powder in a dish. After I had flushed the
powder down the toilet, I felt much better.

Sylvia looked very upset when she saw her evening
bag. I don't think she recognised it at first.

* * *

I now spend a great deal of time in the garden. It is so peaceful as I potter among the plants.

Early one morning, I decided to mow the lawn and went into the shed to get out the motor mower. There was an old spade on top that I removed, but before I put it down, I stared at it. It surprised me how rusty it had become because of lack of use.

I noticed that Sylvia's smaller spade was bright and clean. She must be digging the garden regularly now.

That used to be my job.

After mowing the lawn, I forgot all about the rusty spade and went back into the house. Sylvia was not up yet so I went into my den and sat at my computer. I intended to write up my diary. Sylvia came in and asked how I was getting on. 'Not started yet, just about to get going,' I mumbled.

'Oh, but you've been in here all morning. It's nearly time for lunch.'

'What time is it?'

'12.30. Lunch will be ready in half an hour. I'll give you a call.'

When she had left, I looked at the empty screen I had been staring at for three hours. I had not even opened my word processor progam yet.

I remained in the root directory and idly played about with the keyboard.

'What am I going to do?' I typed.

'Bad command or file name,' the screen flashed.

'I know, I know!' I typed. 'If you're so smart though, why haven't you got any answers to a REAL problem?'

'Bad command or file name,' the computer replied.

'You may be one of the fastest and most powerful computers in the neighbourhood,' I typed, 'but ill as I am, I'm a hundred thousand times smarter than you.'

I switched it off in disgust before it could say bad command or file name again and went in to lunch.

* * *

We went to the cinema yesterday evening and I am afraid I embarrassed Sylvia towards the end of the film. (Amendment: she has just told me it was during the whole film, and not just at the end.)

Although her arthritis was troubling her, she drove us in the car as it is only a few kilometres. The film was *Sleepless in Seattle* which we both found very moving. However, several scenes proved a bit TOO moving for me and I burst out sobbing near the end. I have never cried in the cinema before, or anywhere else, from my childhood to the time I became ill.

It would not have been so bad if I had just wept quietly to myself, but these were deep heart-rending sobs that caused everyone to look round. One or two people shouted for me to be quiet, but most of them just laughed and pointed. Several youths started to clap and cheer while urging me on to greater efforts.

Sylvia just stared straight ahead and sank down in her seat. She seemed really put out by it, but I did not care what anyone thought and kept on sobbing.

One side-effect of this illness, about the only one that is not unpleasant, is that I seem to have lost all sense of embarrassment and just do not care what other people think. I kept sobbing loudly even after the film was over and we walked out among the crowd. I felt that it was doing me good; in some way, it seemed as if it was a catharsis and I felt much better for it.

At first, I did not suppose we would be going out again for a long time. However, while we were walking away from the cinema, Sylvia suddenly paused and doubled up holding her sides. For a second, I thought she was ill, then I realised that she was laughing uncontrollably.

'What's so funny?' I asked.

'Oh, the way those lads were egging you on, and you sobbing your heart out. I'm sorry. I shouldn't laugh, but it did strike me as funny.' She wiped her eyes, and continued, 'I know you couldn't help it, dear, and I'm sorry for laughing. There, I'm better now. Oh, oh!' She was off again, and this time I joined in.

We stood there holding each other, giggling and spluttering together, while the passing crowds gave us a wide berth.

* * *

On re-reading what I have written to date, it seems to have been one event or calamity following fast on the heels of another. Of course, it was not like that at all.

These recorded events are just the ones that stand out sufficiently for me to remember. Or more often, the ones that Sylvia reminds me about. The time span, which encompasses several years, therefore seems compressed in the story.

Another side that I seem to have over-emphasised is Sylvia being upset about some of the things I did. Most of my actions caused us to burst out laughing together, as we did outside the cinema. Although I have a dreadful illness, it does have its lighter moments. Sylvia and I have always laughed a lot together, but we both seem to find even more to laugh at lately . . . I suppose it's just as well really. If we did not laugh so much, perhaps we would cry.

My memory loss and other symptoms seem to fluctuate, and with it my progress with this story. Sometimes I do not write for many days, or even weeks, and then one morning I feel better and begin writing again.

Of course, the first thing I have to do is correct all the bad grammar and spelling that have gradually deteriorated as my condition worsened. My fluctuating condition reminds me of a day I spent on the seashore as a child. We lived in Southport for a short while.

In my mind I was back there now, walking down the seemingly never-ending beach to the distant sea. I stood there watching the tide come in, and tried to observe a pattern in the movement of the waves.

As they lapped against the shore, I noticed that every seventh wave was larger than the rest. I started counting and sure enough they were all in multiples of seven, with wave number 49 a little larger than number 7. (I thought that number 343 wave – being 7×49 – should be still larger, but of course it was not. I waited for one but I could not see any difference in size before the tide started to go out again, so I went home.)

My periods of lucidity seem to progress in much the same fashion. I am on a plateau of incomprehension that clears a little from time to time as the waves recede; and occasionally, it clears dramatically for a short while and I am almost my old self. This is the case now, and I can think with welcome clarity. I will try to write as much as I can before the tide of fog again returns. (By the way, I now know the reason wave number 343 was no larger than number 49. It's because I multiplied 49×7. I think I should have squared it. Would anyone like to go out and see if wave number 2401 is larger than the rest?)

* * *

I have never been an avid viewer of television, but I used to enjoy a good film occasionally. Now I find I just cannot follow the plot.

I would sit desparately trying to concentrate, but find my mind wandering or going into a stupor. Sometimes,

I tried to concentrate so hard that I ended up not watching the film at all.

I just sat there thinking to myself, 'Now concentrate, I really must concentrate on the film', then coming to with a start and realising that half an hour had passed without me looking at the screen. I think the trouble lies within my short-term memory. I seem to forget an incident on the screen within a few moments of viewing it.

There is an advantage to this. There cannot be many viewers who can watch both the original screening and the weekly repeats of 'Coronation Street' with such a fresh interest.

I really will have to think about doing something to improve my short-term memory.

It's the same with books, but to a much lesser extent. At least, I can go back over the earlier chapters to enhance my understanding. Sometimes while I am writing this, I find that I have repeated something I said only a few lines earlier.

It's as though I have already forgotten I have just written it. I think the trouble lies within my short-term memory. I seem to forget an incident on the screen within a few moments of viewing it.

I really will have to think about doing something to improve my short-term memory.

I do not know how I would manage without Sylvia. She is very understanding but has to put up with so much. She seems to make allowances for me because of my illness.

No, that's not right. I think she has ALWAYS made allowances for me.

I did not know how lucky I was in my choice when I married her. When we met, I didn't think she was interested in me at all: I thought it was my motorcycle she fancied.

If it was, then I am glad I bought it!

One day, Sylvia must have heard me groaning because she came running in from the kitchen. 'What's the matter, chucklychops, are you all right?'

'No, I've got a flaming headache.'

'Oh, I'll get you something for it, I won't be a moment.'

I held my pounding head. It seemed ages before she returned with a blister pack of tablets and a glass of water. She popped a couple of tablets out, then put the blister pack on the coffee table beside me, and handed me the tablets.

I swallowed them with a sip of the water.

I sat there after she went back into the kitchen, waiting for the pain to subside. I noticed an aroma from the kitchen door. 'Chicken soup!' I thought. I loved Sylvia's chicken soup. My mother used firmly to believe that hot chicken soup could cure all ills.

The pain in my head seemed to be getting worse.

I used to suffer with migraine headaches, and once even knocked myself out by banging my head on a wall. As I approached middle age, they eventually stopped and it is many years since I have had a headache as bad as this.

I leaned forward to relieve it and noticed a packet of painkillers and a glass of water beside me. They were not my old Migraleve tablets, but they still might do the trick. I took a couple of them and a sip of water and noticed that the smell of soup was getting stronger. 'Won't be long till lunch now,' I thought, 'or is it tea time?'

I never seemed to know what time it was lately. I looked at the clock. Sometimes I could still tell the time, while at other times, the clock face seemed to have no meaning for me. I squinted at it, but it made my head worse. I had a terrible headache, but fortunately there was a packet of painkillers and a glass half-full of water on the table beside me. I took a couple of tablets and a sip of water. I hoped they would not take too long to work.

The throbbing in my skull made me screw up my eyes in pain. My eyes began watering, and I felt in my pocket for a handkerchief. As I wiped my eyes and blew my nose, I noticed a smell of chicken soup coming from the kitchen. Through a crack in the door, I could see a woman in there cooking the soup in a small saucepan. It did not look like my mother, but who else could it be? She had her back to me, but I could tell by the smell that dinner would not be long. I had a bad headache, and noticed that Mummy had left some tablets for me. I took two of them and had a drink of water. I hoped Daddy would come home soon so that we could have dinner. Mummy never put it on the table till he came home. Mummy knew he got cross if his dinner was cold. The pain in my head was getting worse. There was a packet with two tablets next to me. I know Mummy always takes tablets when she has a headache. She must have left these for me. I put the tablets in my mouth, but needed some water to swallow them with. There was a glass next to me, but that was no good because the stupid thing was empty. 'Mummy,' I called, 'I want a drink of water!'

The woman in the kitchen came running in and shouted at me. 'How many of those have you taken? My God, the packet's empty!' She telephoned someone and a big red and white ambulance came and took me to hospital.

They did all horrible things to me there and made me sick! After a while, I began to feel better and they said I could go home.

A lady came into the ward to fetch me. She told me to get dressed quickly because she had telephoned for a taxi and it would be here soon.

All the nurses waved me good-bye.

I think one of them had a cold because she kept blowing her nose in a big hankie. They should have let her stay at home till it got better.

On the way back in the taxi, I realised that the lady next to me was Sylvia. We were MARRIED!

We went indoors and noticed a burning smell. The chicken soup had boiled dry and the pan had burnt.

Sylvia had forgotten to turn it off before we left. She seems to be getting quite forgetful lately.

I get quite worried about her sometimes.

CHAPTER SIX

Sylvia

*

T his is now written by me, Sylvia. Louis has been
getting worse over the last few months, and I suggested doing some of the writing for him. I was surprised when he agreed so readily. I have had to correct
so much of his work lately that it is now far easier for me
to write it in the first place.

I have to watch him more and more of late. Things
like cleaning his teeth become neglected if I do not keep
reminding him. I sometimes ask him if he has cleaned
them and he swears he has, but when I feel his
toothbrush, it is bone-dry. When I showed him how dry
it was this morning, he said that he had cleaned his teeth
and accused me of drying the brush on the radiator.

We seem to have solved his problem of him not
recognising faces. When we meet anyone, I always
address them by name and look at Louis. I can tell if he
then seems to recognise them and bring him into the
conversation. If he does not, I chat to them about things
he should know about them. This often works, and
eventually his face lights up in recognition. I think
perhaps his problem is not that he does not recognise
people at all, just that it takes him a long time to do so.
It's as though his mind is fighting its way through a
dense fog all the time.

With the disability living allowance, income support
and my carer's allowance, we seem to be just about coping on the financial side, even though I have to pinch
and scrape a bit. Of course, we have had to change our

whole lifestyle. Louis has always been a bit of a gourmet, and although we frequently ate in restaurants, I still used to spend £100 a week just on food.

The three tiny pensions that Louis has will just about cover the extras at Christmas, but strangely enough, having adjusted to a lower living standard, we do not seem to be doing too badly. I think it's because, for the first time since Louis started to be paid on commission, we now have a REGULAR income. Small as it is, I can now budget for a change whereas before, although he often brought home a four-figure cheque for a single week's work, there were the weeks when we were paid nothing at all. Sometimes, he could make several large sales in a week, yet not receive a penny, because unless the customer paid a substantial deposit, Louis did not get any commission until the kitchen or double glazing or whatever he was selling was installed. This was often several months, or occasionally a year, later. Now, at least I know where I stand each week and can budget accordingly. If I save a little out of my housekeeping, we can even manage the occasional treat. However, this can sometimes backfire.

We used to dance regularly in the old days, but recently, when we decided to have a night out and went to a ballroom, Louis could not remember the simplest steps. It's not just that he is rusty; if it was, he would have picked it up after a waltz or two. It was as though he had never learned to dance. It would not really have bothered me if he was having a good time, and at first we certainly were. We laughed so much as our feet became entangled that some of the more serious dancers glared at us.

However, Louis' mood changed as he became frustrated at no longer being able to dance and it eventually distressed him so much that I thought it best to leave.

The following day I found a local dancing teacher who gave private lessons and does not charge the earth. We have been going there twice a week for the last two months. It takes quite a slice out of our pension, but that is not the reason we are giving it up. Louis is not making any progress, and now he is calling it a waste of money.

The first day I thought he was picking it up, and we ended by completing a couple of routines, but on the next lesson, he had completely forgotten them. On each lesson, we have to start right at the beginning, and as I thought the teacher might be getting a little impatient with him, I confided the reason to her. It's not just the steps he forgets; several times when we arrive, I realise that he has completely forgotten ever coming to the place at all. He always greets the teacher like a stranger, and so I have decided that it is not worth going any more.

I will have to buy one of those little dial locks for the telephone. He keeps trying to telephone his mother in London. Of course, he does not remember the number, and even if he did, someone else will have that number now. Even then, it would be different as London numbers are no longer 01 but 0171 or 0181.

He seems to dial at random, and whenever he gets through to someone, he keeps asking them to put him through to her. He will not take no for an answer. It must be adding a fortune to our phone bill. I twice reminded him that his mother died ten years ago, but will not do so any more as each time I told him it came as a fresh shock to him as though she had just died. No one should have to mourn afresh each time so long afterwards. His father died a few years before his mother, but I do not know whether he is aware of that either.

I try to be patient with Louis, but sometimes I feel guilty when it all gets a bit too much.

Like when I have to take him shopping with me, I get so exasperated at having to push and pull him everywhere like a small child. He might act like a child, but really he is such a heavy lump. I also worry about telling him when I have to go out sometimes, as he often throws tantrums.

Then again I have to drop everything I am doing if he wants something, as he has no patience at all. Dr Sherpa told me that I must not argue with him, or raise my voice. I try not to, but sometimes I feel like screaming.

*　　*　　*

Today is Boxing Day and Louis is still in bed. It's very unusual because he normally gets up very early. I think yesterday must have tired him out. Ruth, Philip and our grandchildren came round for Christmas lunch. The house was crowded, and then towards noon, there was a knock on the door. It was Bernard, our next-door neighbour from the flats, whom we had told to pop in to see us when he was in the area. Of course, we invited him to stay for lunch also, and there was hardly room to move in our tiny dining room.

I had a very busy morning, partly because I had to re-wrap all the Christmas presents. Louis was up very early yesterday, and found all the presents I had wrapped and put round the tree. He must have assumed that they were all for him, because I found him sitting on the floor in the midst of them. He had unwrapped them all and strewn the fancy paper and ribbon all round the room. He was happily playing with the children's toys, and had nearly made himself sick with the contents of a large box of chocolates.

I am quite glad that he is still in bed. I have just popped in to see if he is all right and he is sleeping soundly for a change. It gives me a few minutes to have a quiet cup of tea.

Thinking back over the years, I believe that Louis has been ill for a lot longer than I first realised. I remember one evening when he came home from a Round Table dinner.

He was wearing an unusual maroon silk shirt with a red tie that clashed badly with it. I had never seen him with a shirt like it, as Louis normally wore plain white ones.

The shirt did look vaguely familiar though, and then it came to me. It was not a shirt at all; he had gone out in his pyjama jacket. For some reason that I do not recall, he had had the day off work and had worn a turtle-neck pullover. He must have absent-mindedly put the pullover on top of his pyjama jacket in the morning, then taken it off and replaced it with a tie to go out. He used to dress so meticulously; I am sure that was an early symptom of his illness.

He left the Round Table when he was 40, which is the upper age limit for members, so that means that if this WAS an early symptom, it has been developing for nearly 20 years.

On the other hand, some of the things he did might just be due to his poor hearing. He has always been slightly deaf, and although he has a hearing aid, he seldom wears it as he finds it uncomfortable, and as he puts it, 'Not worth the bother'.

He once had to give a vote of thanks to a speaker at a Round Table dinner. The subject was sky-diving, and when the speaker mentioned that he strapped an oxygen bottle on, Louis made a note to ask him in his reply from what height he jumped. There was a stunned silence after Louis gave his vote of thanks. Nobody could understand what he was talking about. Then a shout of laughter went up as one of them realised and shouted out, 'He thought the talk was about sky-diving!'

It had, of course, been about skin-diving from a boat.

I find coping with Louis very trying at times. It may sometimes be due to his deafness; but I am sure that it is often not. He asks me about something, to which I reply, and then he asks me the same question again a few minutes later. Sometimes, he asks the same question six or seven times, and I have to stop what I am doing to answer him. He will not let me reply while I am working. Unless I put down what I am doing and turn to face him, he tells me that I am not paying attention to him. I know it's a problem with his memory, but it's very frustrating to answer a question knowing that he will ask it again in a very few minutes.

The opposite also applies. Sometimes, he expects me to know something that he says he has told me but has not.

He then accuses ME of having a bad memory.

He also forgets the names of things, or calls them the wrong name. He might say something like, 'Have you read the bucket?' He knew exactly what he meant, but used the wrong noun. If I then said, 'What is a bucket?' he would reply, 'You know, the BUCKET. The one that comes through the letterbox every morning.' I would then know that he meant the newspaper. When he used the wrong noun, the word he used seemed to bear no relation to the correct one at all. It also seemed to be the most familiar items that caused him the most difficulty. Perhaps it is because he has to stop and think more about what he is saying with unfamiliar things.

I noticed a peculiar delusion that he seems to be developing. He would slowly bring one hand up to his eye and squint at things past it. Then he would sometimes rush to the bathroom mirror and stare at his reflection. When I questioned him he did not want to talk about it at first; then he told me he was growing extra pupils. I asked him what he meant, and he said, 'I just told you. I'm growing an extra pupil in each eye.'

I thought it best to humour him and just said, 'Well, that will be nice, dear.'

He glared at me and neither of us has mentioned it since. I still see him doing it, but I think he wants to keep it to himself, as he usually does it when he thinks I am not watching him.

He is also getting very possessive and gets lonely when I am out of his sight. It's got to the stage that I have to tell him where I am going before I even visit the bathroom in case he suddenly notices that I am not nearby.

I have to tell him before I go out to the shops, and leave a prominent note about where I have gone and when I will return. While I am in the shops, especially if there is a queue, I begin to wonder if he is worrying or feeling lonely. It makes me feel imprisoned at times.

By the way, talking of the clash with the red tie and his pyjama jacket, Louis cannot knot his tie or do up his shoelaces now. It is as if his fingers just do not obey his brain. He will not allow me to tie his shoelaces for him; so last week, we had to go out and buy him some slip-on-style shoes.

Because he cannot fasten the knot, he does not wear a tie any more. At one time, he would not have dreamt of going out of the house without one, but it does not seem to bother him now. Most people do not wear ties these days so he does not look out of place.

He seems to have lost all sense of direction and cannot even find his way around the house. I am not sure if Louis has already mentioned it, but I have had to put cards on all the doors, with the name of the room on them. 'Bathroom' and 'Dining room', etc. At one time, it would worry me what visitors thought, but these days I have more important things to worry about.

The insurance money for the car accident came last month. It has taken them a long while to pay up. We used some of it to buy another car: a much smaller one than before, a Lancia Y10. It is even smaller than a Ford Fiesta, but big enough for us now that Louis has retired. As we do not have a garage any longer, it stands outside on our drive.

Louis is now getting even more possessive, and sometimes he panics if he cannot find me. This can sometimes be embarrassing. Last Monday, I went to the local post office to buy some stamps. It's only round the corner, so I told him where I was going, and that I would not be long.

However, I forgot it was Monday, and there was a large queue of people collecting their pensions and Giros.

I was almost at the counter when I heard Louis calling from behind me, 'Why did you leave me alone so long. I missed you. Please come home.' Although a grown man, his voice had a childlike quality. He was barefoot and seemed almost in tears. I had to forget the stamps and take him home.

His speech is deteriorating rapidly and he is using simpler and more childish words.

* * *

I found an oil painting in the bottom of an old trunk yesterday. A beautiful monochrome study of Conway Bridge that I thought we had lost forever. When I showed it to Louis, he giggled like a child and said, 'pretty picture'. At one time, he would have frowned if I used the word 'pretty' to describe something. 'That is a very weak modifier,' he would have scolded me, 'can't you think of a more precise expression?'

Now he calls everything 'pretty'.

I asked him if he recognised the picture, and he said no, even though he painted it shortly after we were married.

In spite of what the doctors say, I know he will get better eventually. He told me that he would, and that means he will.

He has always achieved what he set out to do.

He always rises to a challenge. After demob from the army in 1957, Louis became a salesman in a shoe shop. After a few weeks, the manager told him that he would 'never make a salesman'. He has spent the rest of his life proving him wrong.

After a couple of years as manager of one of the largest bespoke shoe shops in London, he left to join Nu-Swift Fire Protection as a commission-only salesman. While most of the others regarded it as a 9-to-5 job, saying that the only time they could work was when the factories and offices were open, he worked seven days a week, from before 8 in the morning until after 10 at night. He took a pride in searching out places that were open at the weekend, and found that many bosses arrived at work early, and he could see them before their secretaries and receptionists arrived to put up the barricades. In the evenings, he called on pubs, clubs and other places that were still open.

Nu-Swift, with a sales force of about 400, in those days had an incentive scheme whereby the top ten salesmen and their wives went on a free holiday each year. He stayed with the firm for 12 years and **always** qualified for the holiday.

He has worked on a commission-only basis for several other firms since, and he constantly strove to be the top salesman in the company. I would have liked him to have taken a job with a regular salary, but as he says he prefers 'to be paid what he's worth on his own results'. He often says, 'I wish Mr Gibson' (the shop manager who said he would not make a salesman) 'could see me now.' Another example of him rising to a challenge is his driving. He always takes such pride in it.

He failed his driving test so miserably the first time that the examiner advised him to use public transport in future as he did not think that he would ever make a competent driver. He promptly filled his car with petrol and went off for a full day's drive, determined that he would be competent by the time he returned. He passed his driving test a month later, and the IAM test three months after that. That still was not good enough for him, so he passed the IAM motorcycle test and later became an examiner for the motorcycle proficiency scheme.

＊　＊　＊

I recently thought about selling the car as I do not drive much due to my arthritis. It's just sitting outside the house going rusty. I changed my mind because Louis seemed upset when I mentioned it. He seems fascinated with it and sits outside watching it for hours. I asked him about it once and he told me that he was watching it rust up. I thought that would upset him, but for some reason, it seems to have the opposite effect.

For several months after Dr Sherpa diagnosed him as having Alzheimer's disease, we did not notice any deterioration in Louis' condition. Dr Sherpa said that this was because 'he had started out from a higher plateau than average.' On our first interview, he had routinely asked Louis what his father's occupation was, and he had answered, 'Oh, he was an accountant.' I had to explain that his father was not just an ordinary accountant. He had been a financial advisor to the US Government before the war. During the war he came to Britain and was stationed at Burtonwood as the chief paymaster for the American Air Force over here. I think his title was Paymaster General or something.

After the war, he stayed here as an accountant, and also an inventor.

One of his ideas was to drill holes in the back of boats to let the water out. He said that as long as the boat sailed fast enough, then owing to the lower pressure at the stern, the water would flow out, and not in.

Everyone pooh-poohed it at the time, but after his death, it became a standard fixture on most small sailing boats. He also invented and took out a patent on a type of hovercraft long before Christopher Cockerell. As usual, he let the patent lapse.

Louis follows in his footsteps. One of his inventions was a mechanism to raise the side-stand of a motorcycle as soon as the rider put it in gear. He kept the patent going for a couple of years, and approached Norton and Triumph with it. They said that it would add to the cost and people would not be willing to pay extra for it. Several years later, the Japanese put an identical system on nearly all their bikes. Louis did not seem too bothered about it. He said that as long as it saved kids from falling off their bikes when the stand hit the ground then that's all that mattered.

Louis wrote a short science fiction story many years ago about the Big Bang not being the start of the universe. He told about it being just one in a series of cycles of explosions and contractions. Now scientists are saying much the same thing.

Louis made something once a few years ago. At first, I did not know what it was, it looked so peculiar, but it kept him busy and I left him to it. After a few weeks, he did not seem to want me to go in to clean out the room any more, in case I moved anything or lost an old screw or paper-clip or something equally important, so I left him to get on with it.

When he first began this project, he brought three or four large Meccano sets. I remember he also used to ask the grandchildren to save their lollipop sticks for him. He had hundreds of them; all screwed and jointed together. The thing took him over two years to make and had gears and levers all over the place. Heath Robinson would have loved it.

Louis explained that the man who invented the computer, Charles Babbage, made a sort of computing machine. It was a mechanical computer, as this was before they had electricity. However, he died in 1871, before he finished it, so nobody knew whether it would have worked or not. Louis studied what he had done in the library, and decided to copy it and finish it off to see if it worked.

As I said, it took over two years, and he was always looking for the most peculiar things to use in it. I remember the day he completed it. He took me into the spare bedroom, which was now full of the contraption. I stared at it; it was so big and complicated. As I mentioned before, he had not allowed me in this room while he was making it. It was all so very hush-hush.

'Well, what do you think?' he said as he finally allowed me into the room.

'The place certainly needs a good clean-up,' I said.

'Not the room, the machine.'

'Very nice, dear. What does it do?'

'I'll show you. Ask me a mathematical question.'

'OK, what's 7 times 6?'

'No, not like that, something more complicated.'

'Oh, all right. What's 87 times 43?'

'Well, I meant a real mathematical question, but let's get an answer to yours.'

He started turning handles and pulling wires and things. I am glad that I did not ask him anything more complicated, because it took him ages, but eventually he looked at one dial and said, 'Three thousand, write that down.' Of course, I did not as I had not got a pen.

He went round the back and looked at another dial,

then said, 'Seven hundred, that's three thousand seven hundred.'

Well, it took a bit longer but eventually he finished and said, 'That makes a total of 3741, and that's correct.'

'How do you know it's correct?'

'Because I can work a simple sum like that out in my head. You should have given me something more complicated to do.'

'Yes, well, we would have been here all day if I had. Tell me something, if you could work it out in your head, why go to all the bother of making this thing?'

'I didn't make it because I wanted to know the answer to your trivial sum. I wanted to know if Babbage's machine would have worked.'

'Oh, and would it?'

'Yes, I thought I had just demonstrated it for you.'

'Hmm, so that's what you just did. A bit slow, isn't it? I mean, if you could work out the answer in your head, then so could they.'

'Oh, it's not that at all. This was the very first computer; and I've proved that it works. You can tidy this room up tomorrow if you like. I'll dismantle this and perhaps we'll get a spare bed in case we have any visitors who want to stay over.'

'You mean now that you've made it, you don't want it any more?'

'Of course not. It's not the machine I want, only the answer to a question. If I dismantle it carefully, you can give the Meccano bits to the children's ward at the hospital.'

As I said, all this happened a few years ago. I forgot all about it until recently when I saw a programme on television. A group of scientists had also wondered if Babbage's machine would work, and put together a model of it. Theirs was far more complicated than Louis' as they had copied the old one exactly, whereas

Louis had used Meccano and lollipop sticks. Still, they were ecstatic when they found out that it did work. It took six of them about ten years to make it.

I wish I had known. I could have saved them the bother and told them the answer for the cost of a phone call.

I am mentioning all this to throw light on Dr Sherpa's remark that the progress of the disease might be slower than usual with Louis because he 'started from a higher plane'. The doctor's words, not mine.

* * *

Apart from his inability to write as he once did, Louis now has difficulty with the most basic arithmetic. He cannot seem to add or subtract even the smallest numbers; yet I have seen old correspondence between him and his father that was all mathematical symbols that I could not begin to comprehend.

I should have realised that there was something wrong months earlier. There were so many clues that I overlooked. For instance, before I noticed his problem with numbers, the gas board asked us to read the meter and send the figures to them on a card.

Louis did it, and they sent us a bill for over £1700. Our gas bill is usually about £60 per month, so we were stunned when we received it. I phoned the gas board and they asked me to check the figures again.

We checked the meter and Louis called the figures out to me, which I wrote down and added to the previous quarter's gas bill. It came to the same total. It was a while before I realised that he was reading the ELEC-TRIC meter instead of the gas one, and the figures therefore bore no relation to each other.

* * *

Louis tries so hard to please me sometimes, but like a little child, it usually goes wrong. We visited our son Michael and his wife Andrea last week. I was laughing at an advert for toilet paper in which a small dog pulled the end of a roll and dragged the paper all over the house.

Louis must have remembered it.

Yesterday, I left him at home for a few minutes while I popped down to the shops. When I returned, there was toilet paper everywhere! He had opened a packet containing half a dozen rolls and draped them through all the rooms over the furniture. When I asked him why, his answer had a strange sort of logic. 'I thought you'd laugh about it again. I had to do it myself, because we haven't got a dog!'

A couple of weeks ago, he noticed that I was a bit upset when the mail came. We are now living on a small pension, and several bills had arrived at once. He asked me what the matter was, and I said that it was just something in the mail.

We did not get any post for the following week, and I did not realise why until my neighbour brought round a letter she had found lying on her lawn.

Apparently, Louis has been waiting for the postman, and when he pushes the mail through the letter-box, Louis waits until he has gone, and then pushes it all back out through the slot again so that I won't be upset.

I do not know how much mail has gone missing, but I have had to buy a padlocked cage to put over the letter-box.

* * *

Before his illness was diagnosed, Louis started to write a novel about the Mau-Mau in Kenya. He had never said much about it before, and I never pressed him on it. I do know a bit about the part he played though, because some years ago, I found a book in the library about the Royal Green Jackets. In it there were several chapters about the Rifle Brigade, and it referred to him several times.

I am mentioning all this to show how much he has deteriorated. I have just found a poem he wrote about the frustration he felt in writing his novel. He must have been ill even then, but we never realised it.

I am going to copy it out here.

I'm Going To Be A Writer!

I'd like to be a famous writer, and write a book or two;
Something well known like 'War and Peace';
    That's what I'd like to do.

I'll start on it this morning; I'll begin it right away,
I'll probably be finished by lunch time;
    It's such a LOVELY day.

But first I'll have my breakfast, and do the washing up.
That was a lovely pot of tea;
I'll have another cup.
Right! That's it! I'm ready, now where did I put my pen?
Is that the telephone ringing?
    My word, it's half past ten!

And now what was I doing? Oh yes, I'm going to write a book;
I've still not found that flaming pen;
    I'll have another look.

I suppose I could use this pencil, now what can I write ON?
Ah, here's a pad of paper,
    Good grief, the pencil's gone!

At last I've got my ball pen, pity it's got no ink.
Where could I have put that pencil?
    Let's sit down and have a think.

I really must get started, twelve o'clock's long gone,
I'll write it in the garden,
    But first, I'll put the oven on.

Better to have my lunch first, then I'll have the whole
    day clear;
That was a really splendid meal,
    I think I'll have a beer.

Now just what was I doing, oh yes, getting ready to write.
It's going to make me famous.
    I hope it won't take all night.

I've now got my pen and paper, and another bottle of booze.
I'll sit here writing in the sun;
    But first I'll have a snooze.

Good God, now it's raining, I'd better get indoors.
I really WILL write this blasted book;
    As soon as I've done some chores.

It's amazing where the day's gone. Time for another cuppa.
I've got the whole evening clear;
    So I'll write it after supper.

Hello! Is that the doorbell? Visiting friends are here.
Let's sit round the fire;
    And open a bottle of beer.

We had a pleasant evening, but I thought they'd never go.
I'd better start writing my book RIGHT NOW!
    But then, oh, I don't know.

Bedtime's here already, but you know what they all say.
If you can't manage it just now;
    Tomorrow's another day.

*   *   *

Louis doesn't recognise anyone any more. I doubt if he would recognise even me if he met me in the street. I asked him about it and he says people's faces are, 'like pink blobs'. What he means is that he cannot discern any distinguishing features. There is nothing wrong with his eyesight; I think he sees things but forgets them before they have a chance to register.

He used to be a bit of an expert on faces. I suppose it was owing to the portrait painting he used to do.

He did quite a bit of painting: portraits and such like. He did not use the modern paints but studied the techniques they used in the past. He stretched his own canvases and ground all his colours.

He knew a lot about bone structure, and used to do a party piece where he asked a group of people to write down which side they normally slept on in bed, fold the paper and put their name on it. He would then tell them the answer before he opened it. He could tell because one side of a person's face is slightly flatter than the other. This is the side on which they usually slept. The difference was not normally enough for me to see, but he was always right.

About 30 years ago, the Methodist church in Balham, London, commissioned him to do a picture in the style of Holman Hunt's *Light of the World*. It was a huge picture and they hung it behind the nave. I am a Methodist but Louis is Jewish. I suppose he must be the only Jewish painter to have a painting hung in a Methodist church.

*   *   *

Occasionally, Louis seems almost his old self. At such times, I have to keep reminding myself that appearances are deceptive and he is still ill. Ruth and I took him for a walk yesterday.

He was in the middle of us holding our elbows as we approached a road junction with pedestrian-controlled lights.

'Come on', he said, very authoritatively, 'the lights have changed.'

We both unthinkingly went with him, and a van had to screech to a halt to avoid hitting us. The lights had changed all right, but they had changed to red. It could have been nasty, but when we got over the shock and were safely on the other side of the road, Ruth and I both burst out laughing. It was the way we automatically obeyed him. He had such a tone of authority for a moment. Pour Louis could not understand what we were laughing at, and just looked at us in bewilderment.

We went home shortly after that. After Ruth left, Louis went into his den and I sat down for a quiet five minutes. We have had the usual ups and downs in our marriage, but on the whole, I think we have been happier than most. I sometimes begin to worry about the future, but quickly put it to the back of my mind. One day at a time. That's the way to handle something like this. If this was a fiction book, I suppose I should now say something like, 'Chin up, old girl, put a brave face on it.' I wish it were fiction, or that I could wake up one morning and find out that it is only a dream. Now wouldn't that be something!

* * *

Louis had been bad all afternoon. He had a bit of shock, and I feel awful about it because it is all my fault. I might feel better after I get it off my chest, but I think I should explain it from the beginning. When Louis was writing the earlier chapters of this book, he asked me to tell him of any traumatic experiences he may have forgotten.

I mentioned most of them, then one day while he was writing, I remembered about the time he went into hospital for an operation to cure a slipped disc. I did not want to disturb him at the time, so I wrote a note about it on a slip of paper, to remind myself to tell him about it later.

He said he remembered all about it when I mentioned it, so I need not have bothered.

A few weeks later he had a bad night and did not get any sleep at all. He was dozing in a chair when I went shopping. I did not intend to be long, and thought that he would probably still be asleep when I returned. To be on the safe side, I scribbled a note on a bit of paper telling him that I had popped to the shops and would be back within half an hour.

Unfortunately, my shopping took longer than I expected and by the time I returned, Louis was in a terrible state.

As I have diabetes and other problems, he had telephoned the local infirmary and Birch Hill Hospital to see if they had admitted me. When they told him they had not, he thought that I was so ill, or perhaps fallen into a diabetic coma, that I was unable to tell them my name. He was about to leave the house for the hospital when I returned. He flung his arms round me with relief and held me so tight I thought I would suffocate. It was very nice, but I felt bad when I realised just why he was in such a state.

The note I had left him said, 'I am just popping out to the shops for a few things. I'll be back within half an hour so don't worry. Love you. Sylvia.'

Unfortunately, I had changed my reading glasses for my distance pair after writing it, and had not noticed that I had stuck it on the door with the other side showing. It was written on the back of the old note I wrote to remind him about the traumatic experience and just said, 'Going into hospital for an operation'.

* * *

Louis' eyes have taken on a vacant look recently. Everybody remarks on it, and it even affects animals now.

Dogs and cats seem to regard him as a small child, or perhaps another animal, and follow him home. The only exception is our neighbour's bulldog. I think it may be because Louis no longer notices him. They used to get on well together, but when we passed, the dog bristled and snarled at us.

Over the last few weeks Louis has been getting much worse. He just sits in his chair all day like a zombie. He won't even feed himself now and seems to have forgotten how to use a knife and fork. If I didn't feed him, I'm sure he wouldn't eat anything at all.

He hasn't lost much weight though. I suppose it's because he doesn't get any exercise. I try to make him get up and walk about, but he just slumps in his chair and I can't lift him out. I try my best and occasionally I do manage to get him up and we go out for a short walk. I am keeping on with the diet sheet he prepared before he became too ill. It consists of foods that are high in sulphur, and multivitamin tablets containing magnesium. I do hope that they are doing some good, but there doesn't seem to be any indication that they are.

The nights are so long now as I lie awake worrying about him.

Something happened recently that made Louis very excited. It makes a change because, as I said, he has been sitting like a zombie and hardly uttering a word lately.

We were on our way back from a walk when we came to a crowd watching firemen fight a small smoky fire in a shop. Louis does not like crowds so we stayed on the outskirts. There was a standpipe near us, and one of the firemen ran up with a coiled canvas hose and attached it. The hose straightened with a loud bang as the water pressure forced its way through, and that is what excited Louis. He did not look at the fire scene at all after that, just kept staring at the hose. He would not let me take him away until after they turned the water off and the hose subsided. He then kept moving it with his foot until the fireman disconnected it and rolled it up.

He seems a different person now. He still sits in silence, but now I can tell that he is deep in thought. The vacant expression has competely gone.

I would like to say a few words here about an organisation that has been a tremendous help and support to me.

I contacted the Alzheimer's Disease Society in 1980 when Louis showed his first symptoms. It is such a relief to know that there is someone at the end of a phone line to sympathise and answer your questions. They always do seem to have an answer to a problem, probably because they have heard it all so many times before.

I receive a monthly newsletter from them with news, topics of interest and even recipes in it. When I first joined them, they sent me a cassette tape with information that I still have. I play it from time to time, sometimes to find useful information and addresses, and sometimes just to have an understanding voice to listen to. I am setting it out here in its entirety so that it may perhaps help another person caring for a relative with Alzheimer's disease:

CARING FOR DEMENTIA

Welcome to the Alzheimer's Disease Society.
In this cassette, we will discuss and explain dementia and its symptoms. We will also explain

how the Alzheimer's Disease Society can support you and your family.

The first thing to understand is that you are not alone. In this country, around 600,000 people are affected by dementia; 70 per cent of these by Alzheimer's disease.

What is dementia?
Dementia describes a number of physical disorders that affect the brain. For example, the ability to think, reason and remember. The loss of short term memory is an early and most striking sign.

People with Alzheimer's disease may remember the village or area from which they came; they may even be able to vividly recall their childhood – but cannot remember what happened a short time ago. In some cases, they may even fail to recognise members of their own family.

Sometimes, the patients may believe it is night when it is actually day. Or they may become prone to confusion and wandering. As the disease takes hold, patients become increasingly less aware of their condition. Simple tasks like tying shoelaces become impossible.

Dementia is usually a disease of old age but it can occur in middle age as well. At the present, there is no cure for Alzheimer's Disease or for most other forms of dementia. However, a great deal of research is taking place.

What can you do?
If you are worried because your relative shows some of the symptoms of dementia, then go and see your doctor immediately.

There are many other conditions that can cause this sort of behaviour and these can be treated. Your doctor may refer you to a specialist. If he/she does not, you can ask him to refer you to a specialist as well.

Dementia does not simply affect the patient. It profoundly changes the lives of family and friends as well. Because dementia is both a physical and a mental illness, it causes behavioural and personality changes. It is relentless and its progress is ultimately fatal.

Although this is a distressing illness, there is much you can do to help the person to enjoy life as long as possible.

- Try to be patient and remember that your relative cannot help their behaviour.
  They are not being deliberately aggravating. This is an illness.
- Show love and affection where appropriate.
- Find things your relative can still do. Praise their efforts.
- Help your relative look nice and compliment them on their appearance.
- Talk in short clear sentences and use a reassuring tone and calm movements.
- Make sure they eat a balanced diet and have some exercise each day to stay healthy. Contact the doctor at once if they seem unwell as any illness can increase their confusion.
- Remove hazards such as trailing flexes or unsteady furniture in the home. Make sure medicines or other dangerous substances are locked away and that appliances are safe.
- Find ways to aid your relative's memory. Always put things in the same place. A large bowl for keys, reading glasses or gloves may be a good idea.
- If your relative wanders, they could wear a bracelet with their name and phone number to contact someone if they are lost.
- Find ways to interest your relative. For example, you might talk about the past, look at old photographs, or listen to music they enjoyed when they were younger.

Those of you who are caring for someone with dementia, or have cared, will be only too well aware of the toll it takes on you – of the endless self-sacrifice, stress, loneliness and depression that it causes. Not to mention the huge social stigmas and the financial burden.

A recent survey by the Alzheimer's Society found that 97 per cent of carers suffered emotionally.

We believe that the carer should be cared for.

Try to make sure you have some time to yourself to relax. Do not forget you are not on your own. The Alzheimer's Disease Society offers support for the carer and lobbies parliament for better provisions. We try to educate the public and keep the issue in the public eye.

If you are a carer, we can help you. For example, here in Manchester:

- We have weekly support groups for carers.
- We can talk to you one-to-one.
- We have a monthly newsletter.
- We do case work. This may vary from advising you on medical problems or providing moral support; to helping you claim benefits to which you are entitled.
- We run a drop-in Centre and organise training courses.

If you live in Manchester, you can contact our Branch Office by telephoning 0161 274 4918 or by writing to us at the Alzheimer's Disease Society, Manchester Branch, Rudcroft Close, Chorlton on Medlock, Manchester M13 9TN.

If you wish to speak to someone in your own language, you can do this by telephoning The Translation Department, Manchester Town Hall, Manchester, on 1061 234 3081.

If you live outside the Manchester area, you can obtain information in English by telephoning the National Office on 0171 306 0606.

You may use the following free phone numbers at any time to obtain further information in English.

ALZHEIMER'S DISEASE	0800 318771
OTHER DEMENTIA	0800 318772
ALZHEIMER'S DISEASE SOCIETY	0800 318773
WHO CAN HELP? SERVICES	0800 318774
LEGAL AND FINANCIAL INFORMATION	
	0800 318775

*   *   *

Before Louis got too bad he wrote the poem that heads Chapter 2 of this book. I sent it to the Alzheimer's Disease Society some time ago and they published it in their magazine last month. I read it out to Louis, but he did not remember it. I asked him what he thought of it and he said he thought it was pretty (he calls everything pretty now but he meant 'very good'). I told him that he wrote it but I do not think he believed me.

The Alzheimer's Disease Society is a large organisation with 18 616 members at the last count, split into 164 local branches. There are also 79 support groups. My branch is at Cheetham Hill, Manchester. I would strongly recommend anyone who has a relative with the disease to find the address of their local branch from the head office. Their address is:

Alzheimer's Disease Society
Gordon House
10 Greencoat Place
London
SW1P 1PH

CHAPTER SEVEN

Ruth

*

My name is Ruth. I am writing this chapter because Mum's hands have become swollen from typing due to her arthritis.

I went to the supermarket with Mum and Dad last week while my husband, Phil, took our children to the park. They wanted me to go with them, but I thought Mum needed a bit of help.

It was a bit of a job to persuade Dad to come shopping with us; he did not want to leave the house. However, he came reluctantly when Mum told him that we would not be able to manage the shopping without him.

I was at the check-out with Mum when a message came over the tannoy. 'Has anyone mislaid a confused gentleman, wearing a tweed sports jacket, who seems to have forgotten his name? Would anyone with this gentleman please report to the manager's office to claim him.'

We looked round and Dad had disappeared. 'We'd better get up there, it must be Louis. Can you tell me where the manager's office is?' Mum asked the check-out girl.

We rushed to the office and found Dad sitting there. It was a bit embarrassing really. They were treating him as if he was a child, and one of the assistants had given him a lollipop, which he was sucking. He just smiled when he saw us, and took Mum's hand as she led him away.

I felt my face going scarlet as I followed them.

I suppose I never realised that Dad was so ill until then, even after the day he did not recognise me. It came as a bit of a shock, I can tell you.

When Mum used to tell me stories about the funny things Dad had done, we both laughed at them and I just thought, 'That's Dad for you.' I suppose I thought he was getting like an absent-minded professor or something. I never dreamt he was really ill. Not my Dad.

I took the children (James is 15, Sarah 11, Jacob 9 and Esther 6) round to see him this morning. Mum is in hospital at the moment. Philip, my husband, could not come to see Dad because he was at work. The younger children, other than James, do not seem to notice that anything is wrong with Dad. When I watch them play and romp with him, I wonder whether they get on so well together because he is now near their level.

When I got there, I noticed a big lorry parked outside the bungalow. Dad was moaning that it had no right to park there as it was blocking all the light through the window. Then after lunch, I heard the front door go as he came in. 'Where have you been?' I asked him.

'Only down to the end of the garden,' he said. 'Have you seen my pliers?'

'No, have you looked in your tool box?'

'No, Mum's hidden all my tools, but the nutcracker might do.' Dad always refers to Mum as 'Mum' to me. I asked him what he wanted the nutcracker for and he mumbled that the valve-cap was too tight to undo with his fingers, and went into the garden again. I did not know what he was doing or I would have stopped him. He came back grinning. 'That's sorted him out. He won't do that again.'

'Do what?' I asked him.

'Park outside our house. I've let all his tyres down.'

'You've what? How on earth do you think that's going to make him move?'

'I don't care if he doesn't now. If he stays here, it's because of me, and not because he wants to park here.'

I could not follow his logic, but the lorry was still there with its flat tyres when it was time to go to the hospital to visit Mum. I did not want the driver to see us, so we went out through the back garden and crept along the fence.

I think Dad thought we were playing cowboys and Indians or something.

We passed through Rochdale market on the way to the hospital and stopped to chat with Bernard, my father-in-law. He had one of his legs amputated about ten years ago, and sits in his wheelchair most mornings chatting to people and giving out leaflets for the Jehovah's Witnesses.

Philip's Mum and Dad are both Jehovah's Witnesses, and spend their time trying to convert people. I used to feel the same way everyone else seems to when they knock on the door, but now I realise what a thankless task they have.

Dad used to do much the same when he went 'cold canvassing' to sell fire extinguishers years ago, but at least his firm was paying him to do it.

Anyway, as we were talking to Bernard, I suddenly realised that Dad did not recognise him. Now that was strange, because where Bernard sits in the market most people stop and chat to him, and I would think that half the population of the town knows him. Dad must have seen him and spoken to him nearly every day. Mum says that before he completely forgot who Bernard was, he remembered that he knew him, but could not think of his name. He used to call him Jack or Jim or some other name, anything but Bernard.

I looked from Bernard in his wheelchair to my Dad, and wondered who was the most disabled.

Alzheimer's is a strange sort of illness. When someone is ill, it is normally a time of sorrow. With Alzheimer's, we seem to all laugh together at the funny things Dad does. We are laughing with Dad not at him, but I still feel guilty about it sometimes.

I wonder if Dad's illness could have been brought on because he used to push himself so hard. He always had to try to be the best at whatever he did. His father was the same. He died when he was 86 and that was through pushing too hard. He was walking to the Turkish baths when a woman with a baby in a pram walked past him. He would not be outdone by anyone, so he walked faster until he passed her. This caused him to have a heart attack and he died in the Turkish baths. Dad still has the newspaper article about it, but it has not taught him to slow down.

Mum was very upset when I called to see her this morning even though she knew that there was no reason for her to be. Not about that anyway. What happened was that when she was fast asleep last night, she awoke very suddenly when Dad shouted out that she had 'painted it the wrong colour'.

She jumped out of bed and started looking for a can of paint of a different colour before she was fully awake. Even when she realised that she had not been painting anything and that Dad was just dreaming, she was still upset. She thought he was mad at her in his dream and had told her off.

Dad woke up and told her it was not even her he was dreaming about, but someone restoring an old motorbike.

He did his best to comfort her, but even though she knows that he is not cross with her, she was still upset long after breakfast.

*   *   *

Well, it never rains but it pours. Mum has been in hospital and I have been popping in every day to keep an eye on Dad. It has been over a week since I wrote anything; I have been so busy. Mum went for a routine check-up and they kept her in to do a minor operation. At least, they thought that it was going to be minor, but there was a complication and it took three hours.

She has been waiting for this operation for a long time; but she did not expect them to suddenly decide to keep her in and do it on the routine check-up. She telephoned me to bring her night-dress and things, and to make arrangements for Dad. I now take Dad to visit her every day while the children are at school.

I found Dad's old slippers in the fridge yesterday. I asked him about it and he said he had been looking for them everywhere, and accused ME of hiding them there. He would not believe me when I said I had not put them there, and so I left it at that. I thought it best to throw out the butter and cheese that were on the same shelf, but as all the other food is either foil-wrapped or in packets, I think it will be all right. I cannot imagine why Dad put them in there, but it'll give Mum a laugh when we go to visit her.

Yesterday, I took him to the ophthalmology department at Birch Hill Hospital. He has to go there every six months for a glaucoma test. Mum told me about this appointment and asked me to tell the doctor that Dad might have something wrong with his eyes as he has this funny habit of holding a hand in front of his face, and peering round the edge. I have noticed him doing it several times, but did not take any notice of it till Mum mentioned it. I asked Dad about it but he would not talk about it.

When I told the doctor that Dad thought he was growing an extra pupil in each eye, he just smiled at me, but after the examination, he told me what it was all about. If you look at an object with both eyes open, and slowly put something over one eye, there is a double outline of the object that changes to a single one as one eye is covered. Dad had noticed this happening even if he kept one eye closed all the time. He normally needs glasses for distance, but found that he could see things a few metres away if he half-covered one eye. He thought it must be because he was growing another pupil in his eye, and was covering it up with his hand!

The doctor explained to both of us that it was a natural effect called a 'pinhole phenomenon'. This seemed to relieve Dad, and I also have managed to do it myself. It's true, if you are looking at something a short distance off with one eye closed, and half-cover the other eye up, there is a position where everything suddenly becomes clearer. Do not do it at a bus stop as I did though, or everyone will start to give you a funny look.

I told Mum what the doctor said about it, and she said, 'Well, I wish everything he does had such a simple explanation.' I am glad that she will be coming out tomorrow because Dad misses her terribly.

After the hospital visit yesterday I met Mrs Hewitt, one of our neighbours, while we were waiting at the bus stop to come home. She was the first in the queue, and we were next, when a crowd of youngsters came into the shelter behind us. Dad glared at them as they started making a bit of a ruckus. It was only high spirits, but Dad is always going on about there not being any discipline these days, and how children had to respect their elders when he was a boy. They had 'to be seen and not heard'. That's what he is always saying.

Well, of course the children did not take any notice; in fact they got noisier than ever. I was in conversation with Mrs Hewitt and we did not notice when the bus came, so the children started to push past us. Dad put both his arms out at the bus entrance and shouted at them, 'Just a moment, have a bit of respect, we are in front of you, and this lady is first.' He turned to Mrs Hewitt and waved her on the bus like an old-fashioned gentleman does in films. 'After you, Madam,' he said.

'Oh no, that's not my bus thank you,' she said.

I looked up and tried to pull Dad back, but it was too late and he was already getting on.

'Where are you going then?' the driver asked.

'Into town please,' said Dad.

'Not on this bus, you're not, mate,' said the driver. 'This is the school bus.'

Well, of course Dad had to get off and let all the children on the bus. Some of the children were pushing past him to get on while he was trying to get off and they were getting in his way. I think they did it on purpose.

It would not have been so bad but the bus was a bit early and waited at the stop for a few minutes before moving off. All the children on the bus crowded to the windows and poked their tongues out and made faces at Dad. He did not seem to notice, but just kept looking straight ahead. I was a bit embarrassed, I can tell you.

We had a bit of a laugh this morning. I made some chopped liver and popped it into the fridge for Dad to have for his supper tonight. He came into the kitchen for a glass of water, then suddenly started hurriedly searching through all the cupboards. 'What are you looking for?' I asked him.

'The fly killer. I just saw a beetle go under the fridge when you put something in it and shut the door.'

'Nonsense,' I told him, 'there aren't any beetles in this kitchen.'

'Well, I just saw one. Or it might have been a cockroach.' He found a spray-can and squirted its contents under the fridge. 'Look, there it is!' he shouted. Sure enough, something small and dark came scuttling out from under the fridge as he sprayed it.

'Stop a minute and I'll get it,' I said as I reached for the broom.

I noticed a fragrance and looked at what he was holding. It was lavender furniture polish. 'It's no good using that,' I told him, 'it's not fly spray but polish.'

He would not listen to me but kept spraying at whatever it was on the floor. The more he sprayed the more it scuttled away, until eventually the can gave a sizzle and stopped as it was empty. The thing on the floor also stopped. 'Killed it!' Dad shouted. 'It's dead now all right. We'd better get an insect killer to put round everywhere in case there are any more of them.'

'Yes, I suppose you've polished it to death,' I bent down to see what it was, then grinned at Dad.

'We don't need to bother about the others. I don't think it's got any little children or anything. It's a bit of liver you've been blowing all over the place with that spray can.'

I stayed with Dad from before lunch until yesterday evening. We had a bit of a problem after tea when it began to get dark. I turned the light on in the lounge and started to draw the curtains. Dad shouted at me to stop as there was a man out there peering in at us. I looked, but could not see anybody. I got a bit worried as well, because the lounge faces out over the back garden and it has a wall all round it. If there was someone out there, he must have climbed over the garden gate, which has a bolt on the inside, and be up to no good. I did not want to phone the police just on Dad's say-so, but did not know what else to do. I thought it better to draw the curtains and was just about to do so when Dad shouted that he was there again, and had brought a woman with him.

I still could not see anyone, and then I realised that Dad was looking at our reflection in the glass. Dad was frantic, but as soon as I turned the light off, and the reflection disappeared, I think he realised his mistake.

He did not want to admit that he was wrong, I do not ever remember him doing that, but he went out of the lounge muttering about people invading his privacy. I stayed a little longer until I was sure he was all right.

* * *

A few days ago, I noticed that Dad was still wearing the same shirt he wore the day Mum went into hospital. I tried to find him a clean one, but there did not seem to be any. I could not believe how few clothes he had. Hardly any shirts or socks or anything. I asked him which drawer he kept his underwear in, and he showed me; but it was empty.

When I went to visit Mum in hospital, I mentioned it to her, and she said, 'Nonsense; he has plenty of clothes. Perhaps he has hidden them or something.' The next day, I searched the whole house, but I could not find anything other than an old shirt and a few pairs of socks.

I was going to wash them for him, when he noticed what I was doing and said that he had some old pullovers and pyjamas that needed doing.

'Bring them in here and I'll do them at the same time,' I told him.

He came in with an armful of old clothes, but still no shirts or socks. I do not know where he kept all the pullovers and cardigans he brought in; I did not see them when I searched for his shirts.

"Why don't we take it to the laundry thingy on the corner?' he asked me. 'Sylvia always does.'

'Well, some of it is hand wash only,' I told him, 'although I suppose we could take this lot.'

I sorted it into two piles, left the hand wash ones to soak, and we took the others to the nearby launderette, or laundry thingy as Dad insisted on calling it.

I put his stuff into a machine while Dad sat on the bench against the wall. I had never used this launderette before, but Dad obviously had.

When the woman who ran the place came out from the back, she took one look at Dad and called out, 'So there you are! I've been waiting days for you. Good job I saw you bringing your stuff in; you're lucky it wasn't pinched.'

I did not know what she was talking about, and neither, it seemed, did Dad.

She went into the back of the shop and came back with a huge laundry bag full of Dad's clothes.

It seems that Dad collected all his clothes together the day after Mum went into hospital, and took them in to be cleaned. He must have put them in the machine and then walked off without them. Luckily, he had a bit of trouble with the machine and the woman in charge had to show him how to use it, or she would not have noticed who had left them behind.

She remembered Dad because he often came in with Mum, but she did not know his name or where he lived.

Mum will want to know what Dad's been up to while she was away. I have got something to tell her that should make her laugh.

Talking about Dad leaving his washing behind reminds me of the story about my Grandad Blank. I see that Mum has already written about him, and I am surprised that she did not mention the launderette he opened.

He was a very successful accountant and had a practice in London with some famous people as clients. Then one day he noticed the new launderettes that were springing up all over the place. This was when Dad was about 11.

Grandad sold his practice and took all the family to Dun Laoghaire, near Dublin. There were no launderettes anywhere in Ireland at the time, so Grandad thought that it was an ideal time to open the first one in Ireland. He found an ideal site, a large corner shop in the centre of the town.

The business would probably have been a roaring success if he had opened it a few years later, but Grandad was a bit ahead of his time. They didn't have many customers and we soon realised why when Grandma told him about a conversation she had overhead while standing at a bus stop outside the shop. One Irish lady had turned to another as they passed the shop and remarked, 'Hmm, fancy having to shop to do your laundry; you won't catch me going in there. I do all my laundry at home. You won't catch me washing my dirty linen in public.'

Perhaps that is where that saying first originated.

✳   ✳   ✳

I am glad for both of their sakes that Mum is being discharged tomorrow.

They both miss each other terribly. Mum asks about every detail of what Dad has been doing at home, when all the time he just seems to sit around pining for her. Still, he seems a bit more cheerful now he knows that she will be home in the morning. I suppose I had better stop writing now and start getting the place tidy for her.

✳   ✳   ✳

This morning Dad seemed at a bit of a loose end so I suggested playing a game of chess. Dad has always been a good chess player and used to be in the local chess club and played in tournaments. He taught us all how to play years ago, but none of us could beat him even though he played without his queen or knights. Today when we were playing he seemed deep in thought after the first move. I thought at first he was plotting some deep strategy, but then I realised he had forgotten how the pieces moved. I tried to show him but he couldn't get the hang of it at all so we ended up playing draughts instead.

There is something that happened during the time I was looking after Dad that I think I should mention to Mum as it may be relevant to his condition.

He had a couple of bad headaches while I was with him so I gave him a couple of aspirins as that was all I could find that was suitable. He used to suffer with migraine and took Migraleve tablets for them but he told me that these are not the same sort of headache. During one of his headaches, he told me that they were a new type of throbbing pain that caused his head to get a hot spot.

He let me feel the top of his head and sure enough there was a spot on top of his crown that felt really hot to the touch. I've never known anything like it. It wasn't just warm as someone's forehead might be if they had a fever, but really HOT.

We had a telephone call from a lady at the Alzheimer's Disease Society this morning. She asked to speak to Mum, and when I told her I was looking after Dad because Mum was in hospital, she asked how I was managing and gave me a few tips. Apparently, she phones Mum at regular intervals to keep tabs on how Dad is doing.

I've got to go now as I have to take Mum's clothes to the hospital and bring her home.

CHAPTER EIGHT

Louis Again

*

Hello, it's me, Louis. The tide of fog has receded and I am writing again.

I have read over what Sylvia and Ruth have written, and wanted to delete some of it and change other parts, but Sylvia has persuaded me to keep it as it is. This is difficult because there are some phrases and words that they have written that really irritate me. Take the section where she says, 'Louis has been bad all afternoon. He had a bit of a trauma, and I feel *awful* about it because it is all my fault.' That word 'awful' that many people use when they mean bad or horrible really means 'full of awe'.

Now I do not think Sylvia was full of awe about me at all.

On the other hand, I may be mistaken.

Yes, I think I will leave it as it is.

As she pointed out, apart from correcting grammar and spelling, she has left my work alone, so I should not alter hers or Ruth's. It seems that what I originally intended as my work has become a joint venture, so from now on, whoever is writing will just insert their name at the change point.

As you may have gathered, I am much improved now. It's early days but I think that I may have succeeded in curing myself. It's been a long and tiring process, and while it may have worked for me, it might not work for anyone else. I hope and pray that it does.

First of all, it's taken a fairly long time. It was several months ago that we saw the shop fire. It was the hosepipe that gave me the idea that seems to have brought about my improvement.

That and a couple of other things.

The rusty spade in the tool shed, and my car rusting up on the drive, for instance.

Both of them decaying through lack of use.

I realised that I had been on the wrong track entirely when I tried to fight the formation of plaques and tangles. They were not the cause of the problem, merely a symptom of it.

I now believe that there is a much simpler and more basic answer, and was surprised that none of the books I had read mentioned it. Then I realised that eminent as the authors were, they had not experienced the disease at first hand as I had.

It's extraordinary how the prospect of a terminal illness can sharpen the mind.

I knew exactly what I would have to do; it was as though I had awakened from a long, drug-induced dream.

When I saw how easily the water pressure untangled the twisted hose, I wondered if a sustained period of intense concentration might have a similar result on the neurofibrillary tangles in my brain.

Also a period of intense thought might have a beneficial effect on the plaques covering the brain's surface.

I believe that the main detrimental effect that the disease causes is mental lethargy. Similar to, but far less intense than, the sleeping sickness that I witnessed in Africa so many years ago.

This lethargy itself is the danger.

I believe that as a muscle that is not in use will atrophy, so when the function of the brain diminishes, plaques form on its surface and the nerve fibres become entangled. If I could constantly force the neurones in my brain to fire, the tangles should straighten just as the hosepipe did. Perhaps the plaques would diminish also.

I recall a fascinating fact about Albert Einstein and his grand-daughter, Evelyn. Dr Thomas Harvey kept the brain that he removed during Einstein's post-mortem, and subsequently sent several sections away for analysis. This showed that Einstein's brain had far more than the average number of glial cells per neurone.

There were other genetic differences, and when Evelyn donated a small portion of her skin for genetic research, it showed that she had similar characteristics.

This was the result that everyone expected, except for one thing. Evelyn, the supposed grandchild of Einstein, is not a blood relative. Her mother was Einstein's ADOPTED daughter.

The scientists are busy trying to prove that in some way she IS a blood relative, but I think there may be another explanation for the similarities. As the last living relative of such a genius, surely there was a tremendous social pressure on her to behave and think as such a granddaughter should. Perhaps with only normal mental capacity to start with, she constantly exercised her brain and this is what caused the increase in glial cells and the other similarities with Einstein's brain.

In the book by Sharon Fish, *Alzheimer's – Caring for Your Loved One,* there are two items that I found of interest. The first is that the brains of people with Alzheimer's do not appear to have the enzyme *choline acetyltransferase* that is present in normal brains. This is needed to manufacture a neurotransmitter called *acetylcholine.*

Therefore, not having the choline acetyltransferase, they do not have the normal supply of acetylcholine either. The nerves in the brain require neurotransmitters to transmit messages. When they are not able to transmit messages, they atrophy through lack of use.

The plaques on the surface of the brain are composed largely of dead tissue, and I think that perhaps this tissue could be the remains of these atrophied nerve cells. I wondered if there are any methods of obtaining or synthesising either choline acetyltransferase or acetylcholine, but could find no evidence of research into this in the books available to me.

The second item I read about in Sharon Fish's book concerns the neurofibrillary tangles and the plaques. It seems that people with Down's syndrome also exhibit both of these symptoms.

I wonder if there is a link there?

I have also read somewhere that our brains have so much unused and excess capacity that there is only a marginal difference between the brain of an imbecile and that of a genius.

In other words, even a genius uses only a small portion of his or her brain's capacity; and it takes about 95 per cent of this used amount just to allow an imbecile to function.

It is the other five per cent that makes all the difference.

Many people believe that *Homo sapiens* achieved dominance because of his superior brain power, but I think that our adaptability combined with the use of technology is the reason. If brain power alone makes us supreme, then judging by the way standards have diminished just in my lifetime our race is in for a swift decline.

Among other animals, dolphins have brains that exceed ours, and we are not even the most intelligent biped there has been. Cro-Magnon man had a far larger brain than *Homo sapiens,* and we cannot derive any satisfaction from the fact that he is extinct while we are not.

Cro-Magnon existed for a period many times longer than *Homo sapiens* has to date, and it could perhaps be the very size of his brain that caused his extinction. Babies were born with such enormous brains that the birth itself was so difficult that it often resulted in the death of both mother and child.

That is why I believe that the size or condition of the brain is not the main factor in intelligence.

It's the willingness to use what we have that counts.

What I have to do is keep my brain active. No, more than that, I have to build it up with exercise in the same way that a body-builder builds up his body. Yes, I liked that as an example and set up a similar exercise routine.

It is fortunate that I never needed the amount of sleep that others seem to require, as I now needed every waking moment I could spare. I began the following periods of mental exercise:

Each morning, I counted down from 1000 in sevens. If the final answer came to anything other than six I began again until I got it right. (After a few days it became too easy so I started with 10 000 as the base number. This time the correct result at the end was four.)

I had a quick breakfast and then started to exercise my memory by memorising poetry. The first poem I dealt with was Macaulay's *Horatius*. I chose this first because there is no better work to set the adrenaline pumping, and secondly it is the longest poem in my library. I learnt ten verses by heart every day, and by a useful coincidence its length is 70 verses. At the end of the first week, Sylvia could open it at random and read aloud any three consecutive words. I could then recite the poem word-perfect from there. I could not have been more fortunate in my first choice of poem. I found the following lines very moving, and bearing in mind the pressure exerted by the water in the fireman's hose, particularly applicable to what I hoped to achieve. It describes the events after the Romans demolished the bridge over the River Tiber:

> But with a crash like thunder,
>   fell every loosened beam,
> And like a dam, the mighty wreck,
>   lay right athwart the stream,

and continuing in the next verse

> And like a horse unbroken,
>   when first he feels the rein,
> The furious river struggled hard,
>   and tossed his tawny mane,
> And burst the curb and bounded,
>   rejoicing to be free,
> And whirling down in fierce career,
>   battlement and plank and pier,
>   Rushed headlong to the sea.

I felt that it was possible to burst out of the disease-induced lethargy and rush headlong into a new period of fierce mental activity.

When I had learnt this poem, I went on to *The Battle of Lake Regillus, The Prophecy of Capys,* the rest of Macaulay's works, then started on other poets.

I found a re-awakened interest in poetry and particularly enjoyed *The Slave's Dream* and Poe's *Lenore.* I did not start a new poem until I could recite the old one word-perfectly.

* * *

Several months have passed since I last wrote anything, and although I began my mental exercise with a great deal of determination, I now find it very difficult to concentrate for any length of time. I begin in all good faith, then come to with a start and realise that my mind has been wandering. I think this is a symptom of the disease, as I have never experienced it to such an extent before. It's such a difficult thing to combat. I *CAN* concentrate by thinking of nothing else but concentrating, but then there does not seem to be any room in my mind for anything that I want to concentrate *ON*. A few minutes after thinking about the subject in hand – mathematics, poetry, etc. – I find my mind wandering again. There must be a solution to this problem, so that's something else I shall have to think about.

An unfortunate effect of my inability to concentrate is that the slightest thing distracts me. I find that I lose control of my temper very easily and unfortunately now take it out on Sylvia. I was trying to concentrate this morning when she came in to ask me if I wanted anything as she was popping out to the shops. I flew into a rage and threw my heavy copy of *Webster's* at her. Fortunately it missed, and she stormed out of the house and left me to cool down.

I never used to lose my temper like this. XXXXXXXXXXXXXXXXXXXXXXXXXXXXXXXXXXXXXX (The above was an unnecessary remark inserted by Sylvia that I have deleted.)

We made it up afterwards, and she told me that she realises that it is the disease and not me acting this way, but that does not stop us both from feeling very upset about it.

✳   ✳   ✳

Sylvia talking:

Going shopping with Louis was very exasperating, because he would always assume that he knew where we were going but he was usually wrong. I really could have done with putting him on a lead if it would not have looked too ridiculous. Also to have to push and pull him in the direction I needed to go was extremely tiring.

Another thing that I find extremely annoying is that he has no knowledge of time.

Consequently, I am often asked for a cup of tea immediately after we have just finished our breakfast coffee and before I have had a chance to wash up. Because of my diabetes, which I control by diet, I have to have a mid-morning cup of tea in any case, but he usually assumes that this is lunch time.

I would have thought that even if he was not aware of the time, his stomach would tell him whether it was time for a meal or not, but sadly this is not so. It's not only his mind that forgets but his stomach also. He sometimes ask me what is for lunch a few minutes after leaving the table, or alternatively he will not believe it is a meal time when it is. He so often insists on having something to eat shortly after finishing a large meal that I will have to do something about it, because he is now putting on weight. So much so that none of his suits fit him. Of course, the fact that he is not getting as much exercise as he used to does not help. I know this is only a minor problem compared to some of the others, but it does worry me.

I found his slippers in the fridge this morning. Ruth told me that she once found them there when I was in hospital. I asked Louis about it, and at first he denied leaving them there, but after a while I wangled the reason out of him. He had picked them up and put them on and noticed they smelt a bit. He thought it was because they were going off, so he put them in the fridge to keep them fresh.

Now why did I not think of that?

Another thing that worries me is that I cannot help being annoyed with him at times.

Dr Sherpa told me not to argue with him but to say 'Yes, dear' and NEVER to say 'No', but it is so difficult not to show annoyance at having to drop everything to fit in with what he wants. Such as when I am doing housework or getting ready to go somewhere and Louis wants things done NOW. I cannot say, 'I'll do it after lunch or when I've finished what I'm doing', etc., because he will fly into a rage and accuse me of not helping him.

I used to find it helped to phone my elder sister, Doreen, just to have someone to chat to. I also phoned Louis' sister but did not let her know how bad he was.

The trouble is that the more he shouts and rants, the more I forget what I am supposed to have done.

The good times are lovely when he is very loving and helpful (though sometimes it gets a bit overpowering), but these days when he is ill, they are very few and far between.

* * *

This is written a few weeks later, and there seems to be a dramatic improvement in Louis' behaviour. He is much more 'with it' now. Because he has improved so much lately, I am now finding it very hard to come to terms with the fact that he is now, in so many ways, acting almost normally. I find that I still treat him like a 2-year-old, because that's how I thought of him, more or less, when he had his tantrums.

* * *

Louis speaking:

My mental exercises seem to be working! I have been much better lately. It is only now, after my mind has begun to clear, that I appreciate the dense fog under which I have been living. My agoraphobia has also diminished. I can leave the house and go for short walks on my own now, something I have not been able to do for months.

Tomorrow will be a real test though. We are planning to spend the night away from home. A team of decorators is going to decorate our house, and they have promised to complete it within two days, providing that I am not on the premises.

I would have taken that as an insult at one time, but I know what I have been like recently.

We are going to stay at a hotel in Stockport overnight. We will have lunch and dinner there the first day, and after breakfast the following day, we will tour the countryside, hope to find a pleasant country restaurant for lunch and return home in the evening to a newly decorated house.

It will be such a break for Sylvia, not having to cook or do any housework. She does all the cooking now. She still will not allow me in the kitchen. I am excited about the thought of it, but slightly worried. I do hope that I do not embarrass Sylvia in any way. Fortunately, her arthritis has not been too bad lately, so driving should not be a problem. We are allowing ourselves plenty of time in case she has to stop and rest.

※　※　※

I am writing this in the hotel lounge on my laptop computer. Sylvia is sitting nearby trying to read a magazine, but her eyes keep closing and she will soon be asleep. We had a very pleasant dinner, but perhaps we have both eaten too much, particularly after a large lunch as well. I feel bloated and may stop writing and have a nap myself soon.

This is a very old laptop machine. I did not even know I still had it, but Sylvia found it when she was packing.

It has only an 8086 processor and a 20-megabyte disk, so I cannot run my usual word processor on it. To do so would require enhanced mode Windows, and while I could probably install an older and smaller version of Windows on this machine, there just is not enough memory or disk space to run it properly. At one time, I could probably have fitted a better processor and a bigger disk, but that is beyond me at the moment. Older laptops are far more difficult to work on than larger computers, mainly because of the lack of space and dedicated components. The modern ones are much better: they are designed with plug-in modules, so that anyone can upgrade them without even using a soldering iron. Perhaps I will try and do something about this one when we get back. That should be an interesting challenge.

Sorry that I have been blathering on about computers for a bit. I realise that there may be two or three people somewhere in the world who are not interested in them, but they have always been a passion with me. I probably will not even transfer these ramblings to my other machine when we get home, so may as well continue just to please myself. I find writing helps me to think.

We had a very pleasant journey here. The little Lancia went like a dream even though it has stood outside our house, unused, for months. It started the instant Sylvia turned the key, and hummed along without missing a beat.

We stopped for lunch at a very smart hotel where I disgraced myself slightly. I do not think it was because of my condition; it could have happened to anyone. We both had a duck *a l'orange* and it arrived on larger than usual platters. I stabbed my fork down near the side of my plate, not noticing that the near side edge of my plate was overhanging the table.

Down it went; the whole lot shot up in the air, and landed on my stomach.

The gravy was so glutinous that it acted like an adhesive, and my chair crashed back as I stood up with the plate and its contents stuck to my stomach.

Several waiters rushed over and cleaned me up as best they could. They brought me another portion, and would not accept payment for it even though it was my fault.

Sylvia was very embarrassed.

I have to finish now as the 'low battery' warning light has just come on. If I do not save my work soon it will be lost. We did not bring a charger with us so I will continue this at home. Bye.

*   *   *

Sylvia talking:
Hello, it's me again. I did not expect to be writing any more, but Louis has taken a turn for the worse. He awoke in the middle of the night at the hotel, and when he found he was in a strange room, he had one of his old panic attacks.

I could not calm him and eventually decided to take him home. After hastily dressing and packing, we went downstairs to find a night porter. There was no one about and the front doors were locked.

Louis' panic was increased when he thought we could not get out, but I found a fire door at the rear that opened by lifting a bar, and we left that way. The fire alarm rang when we opened the door and we rushed to the car and left in a shower of gravel.

I do not know why, but I felt guilty all the way as we drove home. We were perfectly entitled to leave. We had paid the bill in advance the night before and it included a breakfast we were not having. I kept reminding myself that we had to leave by the fire exit as there was no other way out, but I still kept glancing in the mirror in case we were being pursued. I felt like the villain in an American car chase movie, and Louis' panic seemed to disappear as, giggling to himself, he urged me to drive faster.

It did not help when he turned round and kept shooting an imaginary pistol through the back window at equally imaginary pursuers.

It was not yet light when we arrived home, and all the furniture was still sheeted up. We slept in our clothes on the bed, and I took Louis out for a day's drive shortly after the decorators arrived. Knowing what he was like, they refused to start work until we left.

I found a poem that Louis wrote while we were in the hotel. Apparently, his computer battery ran out, so he scribbled it in longhand on the hotel stationery. I am sure that he was not capable of writing poetry like this a few months ago, and I hope that it is an indication that he is continually improving. As I think it expresses his hopes and moods, I am copying it out below. I do not know what the title is, or even if it has one. Perhaps Louis will add it later.

The massive gnarled and sullen oak,
    casts afar its dismal shade,
O'er the still and silent pool,
    its shadow haunts the gloomy glade.
Is no sound heard, not the cry of a bird,
    the croak of a frog or toad.

From the lowering sky
    comes not the breath of a sigh,
    To open a sunbeam's road.
The fetid logs of trees long gone
    moulder and decay.
Slow, slow the wood's life trudges on,
    as it wends its weary way.
As many an old volcano
    with imprisoned fury smoulders,
With oppressive reek of rot and dank,
    the oozing mire moulders.
Beyond the mortal mind it is
    to imagine joy and laughter here,
If 'twere gone, there would be none,
    to shed a single tear.

But wait! A shaft of light appears.
    A solitary beam of splendour,
Banishing fears with golden spears,
    causing gloomy shadows to surrender.
And now loud is heard
    the call of many a bird,
    as nature joyously sings,
And from out of the dark
    comes speeding a lark

With a rush of fast beating wings.
Should ones hopes be massacred,
  then from the funeral pyre,
With their demise, fortune will rise,
  like a phoenix from the fire.

Though parched and dry the desert,
  should a drop of rain but fall,
Life would spring profusely,
  abundant overall.
Though cold and bleak the mountain crest,
  with rocky crags and snow,
Comes palest gleam of sunshine,
  and the edelweiss will show.

'Tis nature's will that for every ill
  a cure is near at hand.
Let mortal man, if he only can,
  now learn and understand.

Matters not the depth of ocean,
  matters not the desert's heat,
Nor mountain height, nor blackest night,
  for life can still compete.

So when your mood is darkest,
  when all your hopes are gone,
Then raise your eyes up to the skies,
  for still there shines the sun.

CHAPTER NINE

Mental Therapy

*

Hi. I have just read over what Sylvia has written. I do not even remember writing that poem.

I wanted to delete it or at least polish it up a bit because I do not think it is very good, but Sylvia will not let me touch it.

When I awoke in a strange bedroom, I lost all sense of identity and felt that I had to get home at all costs. I feel bad about spoiling the first holiday away from home Sylvia has had for over a year. It might indicate that we can never hope to go on holiday again. I would not mind that for myself, but Sylvia needs an occasional break, so I really must try to improve.

I am continuing with my mental exercises and, in order to further improve my memory, I decided to write an account of the time I spent in Kenya in the fifties. This would be a real test, as I had not spoken about it for many years. First though, I wanted to learn to touch-type. I had been a two-finger typist long enough, and this would be an excellent way to exercise my mind.

I typed and printed out the keyboard positions of all the keys (numbers and characters as well as letters) and put the sheet away for future reference. Then, with the vacuum cleaner set to collect any dust before it entered the keyboard, I removed all the characters from the keys with a sheet of emery paper. Now my fingers would have to learn the position of the keys and I would never need to look at the keyboard again. I looked at the vacant key tops and made the worst pun of my life. (Sensitive readers may wish to skip the next sentence.) 'Now that's a Louis BLANK keyboard,' I thought.

As soon as I placed my fingers on the keys, I realised that I had made a mistake. In sanding off the characters, I had inadvertently removed the small raised button that indicates the position of the 'F' and 'J' keys. I had to use a small soldering iron to melt a tiny portion of these keys until it formed a tiny blob that I could feel.

I spent three whole days learning to touch-type, and at first I was painfully slow. With two fingers, I used to type at 25 words per minute. Now, with having to find each letter by trial and error, I was down to 2 or 3 wpm. However, it was excellent exercise, and my speed slowly increased. By mid-afternoon of the first day, I was back at my old speed, but now my wrists were beginning to ache. This surprised me as I thought that my fingers, which are prone to arthritis, would have been the problem.

Sylvia brought me in a couple of elastic bandages and I persevered. I practised for 12 hours a day for three days and slowly progressed until I finally reached the target of 50 wpm I had set myself.

To prove to myself (and Sylvia) that I could now touch-type properly, I blindfolded myself and typed out Wordsworth's *Daffodils* from memory. We found a volume of poetry containing it and checked the result. (Seven mistakes – must try harder.)

My fingers were numb at the ends, and my wrists were aching. Sylvia rubbed Traxam ointment in to ease the pain and I went to bed tired, but happier than I had been for weeks.

I awoke at 6.00 a.m. the next morning ready to start my intensive mental routine, as follows:

Memorising poems and writing this book took up my mornings.

After lunch, I spent an hour walking in the park, while rehearsing the poetry I had learned that morning to fix it in my mind.

I then spent a couple of hours writing my book about Kenya.

The remainder of the time I spent writing computer programs.

I used to be able to write in machine code and binary, but now I seem to have totally lost that ability.

I looked at the source code of some other programs I wrote a few years ago and could not understand them at all. Never mind, there was always G.W. BASIC to fall back on. Since this is one of the slowest languages in execution, it is ironic to reflect that its authors gave it the G.W. initials to signify its speed. (Gee Whiz).

Some years ago, I wrote a small sales demonstration for a kitchen company in BASIC, showing a demonstration kitchen with the cupboard doors and drawers opening and closing. Computer people were surprised that I had not used 'C' to write it in, but I chose BASIC so that the user could modify it later.

You are not supposed to be able to draw graphics in BASIC, but I thought that it was an ideal opportunity to prove them wrong. The program I wrote for the kitchen company (using a 'line command' to draw the graphics) was a very simple one.

I now began to construct a more sophisticated program. It was an animated cartoon and I spent two hours a day writing it.

I devised various other mental exercises, and all told spent over 18 hours a day on almost pure concentration. Then for relaxation in the evening, I played a couple of games of chess against my computer. When the time spent on eating and other functions was added, it totalled 20 hours of the 24.

I feel asleep immediately I went to bed, and began

again four hours later.

I began to feel the difference after the first two days. Of course, I was exhausted, but the fog that had been clouding my mind was clearing. After the first week, I reduced my exercises to 18 hours a day, and subsequently to 15, the level I am at now.

I then realised that I had to do something about my physical condition. I had caught sight of myself in the mirror, and hardly recognised the image.

This was nothing to do with my memory. I looked a physical wreck.

I decided to combine my plans for mental recovery with long walks and exercise. During the walks, I continued counting down from 10 000 in sevens, then when I became more adept, I made it more difficult by counting down first in seventeens, then in whole numbers and fractions.

I was aware that people were staring at me as I walked along apparently muttering to myself.

I did not care.

A few weeks ago, I would NOT have been aware of it.

I found that I was able to do things that for the past few months would have been impossible. An example was sorting out a problem on my computer. I still had a small hard drive left over from the time I upgraded to a larger one. Now my drive was almost full.

Rather than use a disk doubler (which I have always been wary of because they compress the contents of the disk into one large file that could possibly be corrupted), I decided to re-install the smaller drive piggy-back on the larger.

To protect my data, I compressed it with a program I often use, PK-Zip, and copied it on to floppy disks. I installed the second hard drive, but when I tried to expand my files, I found the PK-Zip expansion program was corrupt. It is many years since I have used the Boolean code that the program is written in, but now I had improved sufficiently to recall enough to re-write the source code and repair the other faults.

I then attended to another small matter that has been niggling me for months. I typed in some gibberish on the keyboard and pressed 'Enter'.

'Wrong command or file name,' flashed on the screen.

'Right,' I said, 'and that's the last time you'll ever say that to me.'

I altered the machine's BIOS and re-wrote the Command.Com file, and now when I key in an incorrect instruction the screen flashes:

'OOPS, I think there is a chance that you may have made a mistake, Louis, but of course it is more likely that it is entirely my fault. Please try again.'

'A bit more user-friendly,' I thought.

Recalling the trouble I had had trying to make some toast a few months ago, and how I had set fire to it and burnt the grill pan handle, I cooked Sylvia the best breakfast she has had for years. Then I baked some bread and bagels.

It all went without a hitch. Anyone can bake bread at home, but if you want a challenge, try baking bagels. I then cobbled up a new handle for the grill pan out of a block of brass and used the ceramic heat protectors from two old spark plugs to insulate it.

*　*　*

Everything was progressing satisfactorily except for my novel about Kenya, which was not going as well as I had hoped.

I have never had any formal training as a writer; in fact I have had very little education at all. I left school at

15 to work for Monroe Calculators as a mechanic, had a two-day course on repairing calculators, and very little other education since.

We did not have GCEs in my day, and the only exams I passed were for the Army Certificate of Education. My father taught me higher mathematics and such, but apart from that, I am self-taught.

My physical prowess has never been much to write home about either; but recently fate singled me out to show everyone what I was capable of.

Sylvia read about a charity sports day in aid of handicapped people and Mencap, and thought it would be a good idea for us to have a day out to watch it. I had only been out of the house for the odd half an hour lately, and was a bit dubious at first, but she persuaded me to go with her.

We watched several sporting events, three-legged races, egg-and-spoon and such, and I had a go on several stalls. I used to be a marksman in the army, and still have the crossed rifle badge that I wore on my combat jacket sleeve. However, on this occasion I wasted a fair bit of change at one stall without hitting a single clay pipe.

The climax of the day was to be a welly throwing contest, with 15 men from each team competing. I was determined to redeem myself and entered my name for it. A few members from both teams had thrown wellies in competition before, but I had not. Although I have since discovered that it is a well-known local sport, I had not even heard of welly throwing until then.

All the experts were to throw first, followed by the others in descending order of their expected prowess. This naturally meant that I would throw last on our team. That's always been the way.

I have never been a very physical person. At school when the two captains chose teams for football, rugby or cricket, I was always the last one they picked. Then I had to wait for the usual remark, 'Oh, do I have to have HIM?'

As an adult, I had usually tried to avoid team games. My only physical sports were cycling and motorcycling. I suppose I must give off some sort of aura about being hopeless at sports, otherwise why would I still be the last one chosen?

I looked down at my pot belly and tried to pull it in as I lined up behind the others to listen to the umpire as he outlined the rules.

He told us that he would chalk the updated scores on a board as each member threw, and the total of the team's score would signify the winner. I took my place at the back of our line and studied the technique of the others as they threw.

I appeared to be on the winning team. We were so far ahead by the time that the thrower before me on our team came to the throwing mark that all the spectators knew that the conclusion was inevitable. The other team's penultimate man had thrown so they had only one go left. We were 22 feet ahead of them in total, with two men yet to throw. Our man threw a distance of only 17 feet, the shortest throw of the day, as the welly slipped out of his hand prematurely.

That still meant we were 39 feet ahead; until their last man threw a magnificent distance of 51 feet. Still, I only had to lob it over the short distance of 12 feet and we had won.

I picked up the welly and took my stance, conscious that all eyes were on me. At first, I was just going to lob it casually 15 feet or so, and walk off nonchalantly. However, with everybody watching me, I made up my mind that I would show them just what I could do.

I looked round at the crowd and saw that everyone was NOT watching me. Most of them were, but the chap with a ciné camera who had been filming the other throwers had turned his back and was filming the children round an ice-cream van. The last child in the queue had been given her cornet and was handing over her money, so the cameraman would probably turn back to me in a moment. I just had to delay my throw until then.

I looked at the welly and saw some earth and a small clump of grass stuck in the thick ridges of the heel. It had probably picked this dirt up when it landed last time. Anyway, it was definitely an unfair disadvantage so I searched the ground until I found a twig with which I cleaned out the ridges.

The cameraman still had not turned back to me so I began to limber up by running on the spot as I have seen footballers do. The crowd were getting a little impatient, so I put on a bit of a show for them and did some arm swinging exercises as well.

There were a few shouts of 'Get on with it!' which I ignored.

At last, I saw the cameraman turn round and I prepared to throw.

Then I noticed that one or two people, assuming that with such a short distance needed the result was inevitable, had turned round as if to walk away. This would never do.

'Right!' I cried loudly. 'Here goes then.' I knew that this was going to be a throw of a lifetime and I wanted EVERYONE to witness it.

There was a respectful silence and I was glad to see that everyone was now watching me.

I looked at the welly and hefted it to feel the weight. It was a size 12 and a lot heavier than I had imagined.

I fixed my eyes on a small marker in the distance that denoted the best throw of the day. I was determined that I would throw it past there, and in my mind I could already hear the thunderous applause as I did so.

I swung the welly slowly and tentatively in a vertical circle to get the balance, then swung it faster and faster as I had seen the others do. Most of the competitors swung it in two, or occasionally three, full circles before letting go. I knew that if I was to make the best throw of the day, I would need to swing it longer than that to build up momentum.

Round and round the welly went, faster and faster, until I felt my arm pulling at the shoulder joint. I was only faintly aware of the spectators ducking or running for cover when I finally let go. At the last moment, I felt a wrench in my arm as I pulled a muscle, but I did not care.

I was sure that no welly had ever before been launched at such a speed.

Up and up it sailed, higher and higher until it gradually became a small dot in the distance. It paused for an instant, and then became larger as it finally started to descend to earth.

I must say I felt a twinge of disappointment at that point. For one blissful moment, I almost imagined that I had sent it into orbit.

I stood watching the welly descend, then quickly followed the example of the spectators and cowered down with my hands over my head. I had thrown it a tremendous distance, but vertically, and now it was descending straight for me . . .

It did not hit me but fell 15 feet behind.

The umpire called it a minus score and our team lost by 27 feet.

The crowd seemed disgusted and walked off; but one woman stood glaring at me as though I had done it deliberately. When she saw the welly descending, she had clasped a nearby young boy to her and bent over to shield him.

He was eating an ice-cream cornet at the time and it squashed all over her coat. The thing is, it was not even her child.

Never mind, at least I had shown them all what I was capable of.

* * *

The following day we listened to a programme about the Arvon Centre on the radio. It holds residential courses for aspiring writers, and as we listened to the lady recounting her experiences of it, we both had the same idea. It would not only improve my writing, but there would be an additional benefit.

We had our own ideas about what this benefit was.

I thought that if I could stay away from home for a week and cope on my own, it would really prove that I was getting better.

Sylvia thought that if I could stay away from home for a week and cope on my own, it would really give her a much-needed rest.

CHAPTER TEN

The Arvon Centre
and After

*

We both agreed that this writing course could be the very thing I needed and I sent off for a brochure. It arrived within a couple of days.

As I opened it, the first word that hit me was Inverness and I thought that the whole idea was out of the question. Reading further, I saw that they had another centre at Totleigh Barton in Devon, and another just a short distance from me near Hebden Bridge. As I realised that it was within what Sylvia would call a 'reasonable distance', I felt a twinge of my agoraphobia returning.

'Anything interesting in it?' she asked.

'Not really. They've got three centres, one in Inverness and one in Devon. They're both much too far.'

'Oh, and what about the third, where's that?'

'Funny that. Them calling the places "centres" I mean.'

'Why, what's funny about that?'

'Well you can't have three centres, can you. I mean there is only one centre of anything and it can't move from place to place.'

'Oh, I wouldn't say that. You seem to think you're the centre of the Universe, and you sometimes move about a bit.'

'Yes, but there's still only one of me.'

'Just as well. Now, where's that other centre?'

'Place called Lumb Bank. Never heard of it. Must be miles away.'

'Lumb Bank! That's only just outside Heptonstall. Here, let me have a look.'

Sylvia' sudden eagerness disconcerted me. Anyone would think the course was for her. She read the brochure avidly and kept telling me how much I was going to enjoy my stay there. Her excitement increased when she noticed that among the forthcoming events listed in the brochure there was a new writer's course at Lumb Bank that began in only two weeks.

I thought I heard Sylvia muttering something that sounded like 'A bit of peace and quiet.'

'What did you say?' I asked.

'It sounds very good. I think you should try it,' she said.

The brochure showed a picture of a solid stone house set in its own secluded grounds. The syllabus stated that pupils would take part in the running of the house and take turns to cook the evening meal. It reminded me of the holidays that we used to enjoy at Club Med before I retired.

It was a five-day residential course and Sylvia seemed to think that it sounded ideal.

She phoned to enquire if they still had a vacancy.

I crossed my fingers hoping that they had not.

They had.

I felt my panic returning. I realised just how desperately I had been hoping that there were no places left. I also realised that I had been deluding myself when I previously thought I could stay away from home for a whole week. It was only a couple of months since I had conquered my agoraphobia sufficiently to leave the house for a few minutes. I was not ready for a full week among strangers.

'It's a shame we can't afford it, dear,' I said, 'but with

a bit of luck, we might manage it next year.'

'Don't worry, we'll manage,' she said. 'The quarterly pension is due next week and that will cover it. If you think it's what you need then you go on it, darling.'

Sylvia has always stood by me and helped me achieve my objectives.

Blast it!

We drove up to Lumb Bank to have a look at the place before making a final decision. It was at the bottom of a very steep half-mile-long track. There was such a tight left-hand bend just before the house that I wondered how cars larger than our tiny Lancia negotiated it.

* * *

Lumb Bank is an eighteenth-century mill owner's house a mile from Hebden Bridge and slightly less than that from the village of Heptonstall. It is the sort of house that I would have loved to paint in oils before my illness.

The drive through the country on the way back seemed to enliven Sylvia, or perhaps it was the prospect of a week's rest from looking after me. I had to let her down gently.

'It's a lovely place, darling, but we can't manage it just yet. Still we'll book early and make sure of a place next year.'

'Why can't we manage it this year?'

'Well, you can't bring me, you've got a hospital appointment next Monday; and I'm not able to drive yet, not this far anyway. The bus stops at the top of the road and I could never carry my case down that long track, could I?' I rubbed my replacement hip and grimaced to drive the point home.

The sky darkened and Sylvia turned on the wipers as it started to rain. I imagined struggling with my luggage down that slipperty track in the rain.

Sylvia didn't seem to notice my expression, so I coughed and again rubbed my hip and grimaced as I muttered.

'That track's over half a mile long.'

'The letter says you can get a taxi from Hebden Bridge.'

'Yes, but the driver would probably drop me at the top of the track. He wouldn't want to take me down that unmade road; he'd realise that he probably couldn't turn round at the bottom.'

'Don't be silly, there's plenty of room to turn round at the end.'

'Who are you calling silly? You had to a 26-point turn and this car is only half the size of a taxi.'

'Don't exaggerate, it was a 3-point turn and I didn't know the road. If you don't want to go, just say so; there's no need to make up excuses.'

'Oh, I do want to go. It's just that I don't think it's practical at the moment. You know what a nuisance I am at night with my insomnia. If I shared a room with anyone, they wouldn't like it if I was awake reading all night. We can't afford it anyway.'

'Look, I told you we CAN afford it. Tell you what, let's wait till we get home and phone them up. The brochure mentioned that they cater for the disabled. They say they have one private room for anyone who doesn't want to share. We'll tell them about your hip replacement and see if that room's still available. Let's not decide anything until then.'

Our conversation was cut short as we neared Rochdale. We saw our grandson, James, drenched with the rain, waiting at a bus stop and gave a life home. He was shivering with cold.

Sylvia turned up the heater and I passed him a car rug to put round his shoulders.

'Not at school today, James?' I asked him.

'No, Grandad, it's Saturday. I've been to Little-borough.'

I had not realised that it was Saturday, but I do not think that that was anything to do with my Alzheimer's. Since I retired, all days seem much the same to Sylvia as well as me now.

'What's the fascination with Littleborough then?'

'Nothing special, Grandad. I just wondered if I could walk all the way there and back. I would have done it too if it hadn't started to rain.'

Talking to James took my mind off the prospect of being away from home for a week.

Anyway, I did not think it would come to that.

I was quite happy with Sylvia's decision to phone Lumb Bank. I knew that they would not have a private room spare at such short notice.

They had.

* * *

The days and hours until the Monday I was due to leave were a mixture of excitement and apprehension. I went for several walks on my own to convince myself that my agoraphobia was a thing of the past. My metal hip started playing up a bit after its long period of inactivity but improved with every passing day.

I would have cancelled everything at the last moment, but Monday morning itself was so busy, there was no time to think or worry about it.

I dismantled my computer in preparation for taking it with me, then realised that it was far too heavy and decided to take my old laptop instead.

The Arvon Centre had sent me an agenda for the coming week, and one item was in bold type. Pupils should arrive in time for the evening meal, but not before 4 p.m. Sylvia was due at the hospital at noon for a check-up. She probably would not be back in time to see me off, and she suggested that I might prefer to leave the house the same time that she did and look round Hebden Bridge until it was time to go to Lumb Bank. I protested that it would mean spending almost three hours at Hebden Bridge.

I would be much better for me to stay at home until nearer the time, and then leave on my own. 'Don't you trust me to set off on my own?' I asked her.

Her single-word reply of 'No' did not leave me much room for manoeuvre.

I have always known that women just do not understand how to conduct a reasonable argument.

I took the bus to Hebden Bridge. I could have gone by train in half the time, but I was in no hurry and somehow felt safer on a bus. With the stops being far more frequent than on the train, it meant that I could get off any time I wished.

At Hebden Bridge, I found a taxi-stand in front of a converted shop that they used as an office. I explained that I would be calling back for a cab at 3.30, and left my case with them in the office.

Then I had afternoon tea in a cafe. No, I should not have put it like that. I had not been in a cafe alone for over two years. Let's say it properly.

I Had Afternoon Tea In A Cafe.

There were several cafes and I chose a smaller old-fashioned one with Georgian windows, where the waitresses wore traditional black dresses with white frills and cuffs.

I took a window seat and had two cream scones, whose fresh baked aroma wafted ahead of them, home-made strawberry jam, a strawberry meringue and a cup of coffee.

The sun peeked in through the net curtains to make sure that I was enjoying it. I had a walk round the town, then just before it was time to leave I phoned Sylvia to see if she was home from the hospital. She answered 'Hello, darling' on the second ring.

What do you mean "Hello, darling"? How did you know it was me?'

'Well, I guessed you would be phoning. Did you get there all right?'

'Yes, of course. I'm not a child, you know. I had afternoon tea in a cafe. How did it go at the hospital?'

'No problems, I don't have to go back for six months. Are you speaking from Lumb Bank?'

'No, I'm not due there yet. I'm in Hebden Bridge. I've just had afternoon tea in a cafe here.'

'I'm sure you're going to have a lovely time there, darling. Are you going to phone me this evening?'

'Yes, I'll try. I suppose they have a public phone. If not, I'll come back here tomorrow and give you a ring. I'll probably have afternoon tea in a cafe here like I did today.'

The pips went and we just had time to say good-bye to each other. She had not said anything about me going in a cafe alone; perhaps she had not heard me. I made a note to tell her about it the next time I spoke to her.

The co-director, Mark, opened the door at Lumb Bank. He looked very young to be a director of the place. I found one thing strangely reassuring. Mark used a crutch, having only one leg, and the way he gambolled about put my hip replacement into the proper perspective.

He introduced me to Sally, the other director, who made me a cup of tea and then showed me to my room. This again reassured me. I did not merely have a room to myself; I had a whole building! It was a small two-roomed outhouse a few yards from the main building.

There were two beds in it but Mark told me that no one else would be sharing it with me. The smaller room was a washroom and shower. I regretted not bringing my full-size computer. With the desk and chair in the room I could have made it as cosy a workplace as my den at home.

I then had a look round the main building. The nearest entrance was through the French doors leading into the dining room. I counted the places round the large dining table. Twenty-two. There was a huge open fireplace with a full coal scuttle and a wickerwork basket of logs invitingly beside it.

A door at the far end of the dining room led into a comfortable lounge with a similar open fire, and the next room turned out to be a library. I glanced through some of the books and went back into the lounge.

There were two people in there who I assumed were students. His name was David and hers was Kara. I told them I had already looked round the place, and began to describe the library and dining room to them.

Then David explained that he was David Almond, and the lady was Kara May. They were our tutors.

Although we were to prepare dinner each evening ourselves, this first night Mark and Sally would cook and serve the meal. It was an excellent dinner, obviously intended to show us what standard they would expect of us. Reasonably priced red and white house wine was available, and for a house wine, it was very good. Our time was our own after the meal. The writing course proper would begin after breakfast the next day.

The next afternoon I sat a small desk and chair that I had taken out into the garden and began typing away. I looked up as Kara came out.

'Will it disturb you if I do my exercise here?' she asked.

'No, not at all. I'm not in your way, am I?'

I wondered what sort of exercises she did. I did not

want to be too close if she started juggling Indian clubs or something.

'No, you're not in my way. As long as I'm not disturbing you, that's what counts. The writing comes first, you know.'

She started her exercises, which I thought were a type of Yoga at first. She told me they were t'ai chi. I glanced at her occasionally while I was writing and wondered whether I should mention the mental techniques and the exercises I had developed to combat my Alzheimer's disease.

She looked as if she might have understood. None of the doctors had. Even when the specialists had to admit that I was recovering, they would not believe that it was any of my doing. They just said that as no one had ever recovered before they must have wrongly diagnosed it in the first place.

This raises a question. Let's summarise the facts:

1. They are unable to diagnose Alzheimer's except by excluding other symptoms.

2. They can only prove that a person has had Alzheimer's by dissecting the brain after death.

3. The major changes they then observe are the formation of plaques on the surface of the brain and the tangled nature of the neurofibrillary fibres.

If they diagnosed a person as having Alzheimer's disease and a post-mortem showed no evidence of it, they would state that it was a misdiagnosis, no matter what symptoms they observed or how confident they were of the diagnosis while the patient was alive. It was so obvious to them. The disease was incurable and progressive. The post-mortem showed no evidence of it. Ergo the patient had never had it.

Let's look at the situation if just one of those facts was incorrect. Suppose Alzheimer's was not invariably progressive and incurable. If on occasion a patient recovered, the plaques dissolved or were absorbed, and the tangles straightened; then a post-mortem on such a patient who had recovered would lead the doctors to the conclusion that they had never had Alzheimer's.

Could it not be the case that the majority of the patients diagnosed as having the disease, and on post-mortem showing no symptoms, had recovered from it?

That being the case, could not a great deal of the memory loss or 'absent-minded professor' syndrome of the elderly be a mild form of Alzheimer's that was not progressive?

I am setting these thoughts in writing for the first time. I have not discussed them with anyone, especially not the doctors. Once the disease has been diagnosed, they tend to believe that any unusual thoughts a patient may have are merely symptoms of dementia. Come to think of it, who is to say that they are not correct? Perhaps this very thought that Alzheimer's may not always be progressive and incurable is but a symptom of the disease itself?

I still think it strange, however, that the same doctors who admit they do not know what causes the disease and do not have a cure for it are so adamant that what they do know about it is correct.

I now wondered if Kara, who practised t'ai chi and had given a hint in her lesson about her belief in meditation, would have an understanding of the battle I had fought within my mind.

I finished the paragraph I was writing and saved the work to a floppy disk. I thought that if she spoke to me when she finished, I might lead round to the subject of mental therapy.

She paused and smiled at me. I was about to speak when a student came running up. 'Kara, David says can you spare him a couple of minutes in the lounge when you're through? He wants to compare notes or something.'

'Yes, of course. I'm finished now anyway.' She went into the lounge and the moment was gone.

On Wednesday afternoon, I decided to walk in to Heptonstall village. Several of the other students had been the previous day, and told me that there was a pleasant short cut through the wood. This would not only be good exercise for my hip, but would finally lay my agoraphobia to rest. I would have a gentle stroll through the wood, afternoon tea in the village, and then phone Sylvia from a call box. The same call box I had used previously. I recalled how apprehensive I had been that day. And how much better I was now.

I listened carefully as one of the girls gave me directions. 'Keep on this path, but be careful, it can get a bit slippery in places. When another path crosses it in a sort of T-junction, turn right and you'll come out on to a road after about half a mile. Turn left there and it takes you straight into the village.'

The walk through the woods reminded me of the assault course I did in basic training when I joined the army. It also bore certain similarities to the African jungle I was later posted to. I scrambled over fallen trees, trudged through muddy puddles, and once slid down a steep hill that was covered in wet grass, to end with a thwack against a silver birch. I clung to the trunk admiring its silvery bark for several minutes until I regained my breath. I was tired and dishevelled by the time I arrived in Heptonstall. There were no tables available in the cafe I visited last time, so rather than wait, I had tea in another.

A stale cake, and lukewarm tea in a thick mug . . . slapped on the plastic tablecloth by a waitress who obviously wished that she was not.

I idly watched the clouds scurrying across the sky through the grimy windows.

Sylvia was out when I telephoned so I left a message

on the ansaphone. I did not mention about the after-noon tea.

I looked at the clouds and thought about getting a taxi back, but decided against it as it smacked of failure. I had made up my mind to walk both ways, and looked forward to congratulating myself on my achievement when I returned.

I found the path through the woods that had led me here and hurried down it. The clouds were building up and I had no raincoat. As the wood got denser so the path became narrower. It finally petered out altogether. I looked round and realised that this was not the way I had come. Yet I distinctly remember taking the correct footpath at the end of the road from the village.

I then realised where I had gone wrong.

On the outward journey, I had turned left on the path at a T-junction. On the way back, I had passed the smaller path and continued on the wrong one.

I retraced my steps and came to a junction of three small paths. Which one should I take?

I took the right one, which eventually petered out. I went back to the junction and took the centre one. The path came to a dead end at the doors of a barn. There were a few rickety steps leading up to the door which was set a few feet above the ground. It started to rain heavily, and as the barn door was slightly ajar, I wrenched it open and darted inside. There was a scurry-ing from the back that I guessed was from a family of rats I had disturbed. I did not go to investigate as I thought it prudent to wait near the door so that I could see when it stopped raining. There were only two win-dows, a fairly large one high above the door and a much smaller one at eye level that was boarded up.

I wondered who owned the place. It was obviously in regular use, even though slightly dilapidated. Suddenly, the interior was lit up by a flash of lightning. The many cracks and crevices lit up so brightly that the walls for an instant seemed not to exist. The next second there was a thunder-crack and rain beat heavily on the roof.

Apart from the episode in Rochdale market, storms had never before frightened me, as I know they do some people, but this one did. The thunder and lightning persisted, and coming almost simultaneously, I knew they originated almost right on top of me.

There was a tang of ozone in the air, my ears were ringing, and the brilliant flashes of lightning intensified the blackness of the barn in their absence. The rain beat heavily on the roof and walls, and when it paused slightly, I could hear the scurrying of the rats in the brief intervals between the thunderclaps.

I felt a trickle of water running down my neck. The roof was leaking and water was pouring through everywhere. Soon I was as drenched as if I had remained in the open.

I became really worried because, owing to the storm, it was too dark to find my way back, and if it persisted until dusk, I would have to stay here overnight.

This storm was so similar to the previous one – which I believe triggered my agoraphobia – that I wondered whether I would be able to leave the barn when the weather improved. If I could not, I would be in real trouble.

Fortunately, the rain soon eased, the clouds gradually parted sufficiently for me to see, and I had no trouble at all in leaving the rat-infested barn.

The barn was only a few metres from the junction where I had taken the wrong turning, and as I trudged back through the mud, the rain stopped completely as the storm ended.

At Lumb Bank, I was even more glad that I had a room to myself. No one was outside as I went into my little outbuilding, and after a shower and a change of clothing I went into the main house.

* * *

When I came back from the Arvon Centrre, Sylvia cured
me of one of my long-standing problems, cured it as if
by magic with a twist of her hand. I have occasionally
woken at night with a panic attack. I would be in a cold
sweat, fighting for breath, with adrenaline coursing
through my veins. I have experienced these panic
attacks for several years. A few months ago, Sylvia had
read an article in the Sunday paper about a series of tests
that Manchester Royal Infirmary was conducting into
panic attacks and asking for volunteers.

I phoned them and they said that they would like to
see me, so a few days later I went to the Infirmary to see
Dr Miller. She looked very young to be in charge of the
trials, but I soon learnt how capable she was during
the interview. She explained the procedure they used to
study the panic attacks, and as they could not wait for an
attack to occur naturally, they induced them by getting
the patient to inhale CO_2.

I later told Sylvia all about it.

Last week, I suddenly realised that I had not had an
attack for several months. I mentioned this to Sylvia and
she said, matter-of-factly, 'Of course not, I turned the
heating up a bit.'

I thought that she had misheard me and asked,
'What's that got to do with it?'

'Well, I realised the attacks were because you were
cold, so I just turned the heating up and they
stopped.'

'What made you think the cold caused them?'

'Well, not the cold exactly, but I noticed whenever
you were cold you pulled the bedclothes up over your
head. I wondered how you could breathe sometimes,
and then I remembered you saying that they used CO_2
to start the panic attacks, and thought that might be
what was causing yours. So I turned the radiator up a

bit, you stopped pulling the bedclothes over your head, and have not had an attack since.'

I stared hard, and then hugged her.

She had completely cured one of my problems, and had not even bothered to mention it.

A scenario flashed through my mind. Sylvia coming home from the shops and me asking her if anything interesting had happened while she was out. 'No, nothing really,' she replied. 'I just popped out to post a letter. On the way back, I developed a cure for cancer and noticed that the price of bread has gone up by 2p. Oh yes, something did happen though. I met Mrs Jones and she told me her cat's had kittens.'

I do not know whether I will ever regain all of my lost memory. Some things, especially those related to languages, seem to have vanished from my mind.

Other skills are now returning. My sister Valerie phoned me this morning in a panic because she had deleted the DOS directory on her computer. As her unerase program had also been deleted, she did not know what to do.

I thought for a minute. 'Well if you hang up, I'll send you a copy of my unerase program down the phone.'

'Yes, Louis, I thought of that, but it won't do. I won't be able to copy it on to my hard disk or I'll lose all my other stuff. How can I use your program if I can't copy it first?'

'Easy! Copy it out on to a floppy, log on to A:/, and enter "Unerase C:/DOS".'

It all seemed so simple to me now. It would have been impossible for me to solve her problem a few months ago.

* * *

I began doing odd jobs around the house that had been neglected when I came back from the Avron Centre. I was re-hanging a door when the head on a brass screw I was tightening broke off. I searched my tool box for a replacement. I picked up a similar brass screw, then discarded it in favour of a steel one. I paused as I recalled a time when I had watched my father fixing our front garden gate. He had put in strong steel hinges and then had turned to me. 'These hinges and screws will have to be painted regularly,' he said, 'otherwise they will soon rust up. That's your job, so bear it in mind.'

'Yes, you should have used brass ones,' I said, 'then they wouldn't rust.'

'Maybe not,' he replied, 'but steel screws are stronger.'

The recollection of this held a deep and satisfying meaning for me. Alzheimer's disease attacks the memory. Recent ones are the first to be lost, and then the more distant ones. I had been unable to recall any events from my childhood for a couple of years.

Some sufferers seem able to recall long-gone events clearly, but what they are actually describing are the things that they have talked about many times before. This has constantly refreshed the memory, and it could also be that they are not really remembering the past at all, but merely recalling their repetition of it.

This recollection that had entered my mind was a different matter. I had not thought of it in the last 50 years, and certainly not mentioned it to anyone. It was merely a remark in passing that I had forgotten in the flightiness of youth. It now returned with crystal clarity, and convinced me that I am making headway in my fight against this illness.

* * *

Sylvia speaking:
Louis is a lot easier to live with since his return from the Arvon Centre. I am able to do a lot more, like leave him while I go to

shop, though I still automatically leave notes about the house tell-
ing him what time I will be back.

It's so nice to be able to go out together now without any bother
– like to the park or around town or to the library. He seems to be
getting better every day, and is almost his old self again.

CHAPTER ELEVEN

Homecoming

✳

W hen I came home from the Arvon Centre, I decided to travel by train. I would be much quicker, and I no longer felt that I would be imprisoned by the thought of not being able to leave it at a minute's notice. I had not been on a train for many years and now looked forward to it.

✳   ✳   ✳

The journey was a real disappointment. The train had none of the aura of excitement and anticipation that I remember. The carriage was dirty and smelt of unwashed humanity, not the tang of smoke and hot oil that I used to love.

The windows were so grimy that I could hardly see out. Even rubbing a clean spot with my handkerchief, which immediately became black, did not help as they were as dirty outside as in. The seats were torn and uncomfortable and there was graffiti scrawled everywhere. I should have gone home by bus, and cannot imagine why I had been so looking forward to travelling by rail.

These days even nostalgia is not what it used to be.

The train journey gave me time to think about Alzheimer's disease and its consequences. I looked in my notebook for a couple of jottings I had made shortly after I was first diagnosed. The first was a definition from *Encyclopaedia Britannica*:

'Alzheimer's Disease. A devastating and incurable disease.'

The second was from *The Oxford English Dictionary:*

'Incurable, that which cannot be cured.'

I think that one or both of these definitions are wrong. I believe the dictionary definition should have the words, 'at the present time' added at the end.

No disease is incurable: it's just that the doctors do not yet have the knowledge to cure it.

When they do gain the knowledge, the disease does not change its nature from an incurable to a curable one. It's the same disease, but the doctor's knowledge has changed.

It may be only a slight difference, splitting hairs perhaps, but I think it would be far less traumatic for a doctor to tell you that you have a disease that he has not the knowledge to cure, rather than that you have an incurable disease.

I think that the worst thing a person can do when diagnosed with Alzheimer's disease is to give up all hope and sink into apathy. If the person takes action against it, any sort of action that provides some hope and stimulation, then even if it is fruitless, at least they will enjoy a better quality of life while they are doing something about their condition instead of sinking into a morass of despair.

The least action that they should take would be to make sure that they do not ingest any more aluminium.

It amazes me that no action has been taken to prohibit the sale of medicines containing it. I sometimes feel like standing outside the chemist's and shouting at people not to buy them. I know that a few doctors have said that they can find no link between Alzheimer's disease and aluminium. Far more doctors take the opposite view, and I have not read of any doctor saying that aluminium is good for you.

I remember when I was a young child how horrified my mother was when she saw me sucking a penny. She told me that copper was a deadly poison, and I have been cautious of it ever since. Most people are aware of the dangers of lead poisoning, and the authorities are slowly replacing lead water pipes. I think we should be even more concerned about aluminium, the most abundant metal on earth.

I used to be able to speak a few African tribal languages such as Kiswahili, Embu, Meru and Kakwa. These have all gone completely, as have several computer languages such as C+, PASCAL and COBOL.

I try to avoid clichés in my writing. Perhaps here, so near the end of my story, I will be forgiven for a couple. I might be living on 'borrowed time', but 'stolen fruits are the sweetest'.

Dr Sherpa recently told me that while he cannot say that I may not now have the disease, there is still so little understanding of it in the medical profession that he was prepared to keep an open mind. I think he might be trying to say that I may not have it, but does not want to commit himself.

Perhaps I no longer have it, but I do not intend quitting my routine to find out. It could be that I am merely holding it at bay, and it is waiting to strike as soon as I relax.

It's going to have a long wait.

Afterword

*

I now intend to devote all my time and energies, and the proceeds of this book, to funding research into Alzheimer's disease, and would be interested to hear from research centres that could use extra funding. I can think of no better use for the proceeds of this book than furthering research into this dreadful disease.

I have a theory that Alzheimer's disease may be solely caused by aluminium (since I wrote this, I have come to believe that mercury is the worst culprit: see below), and I took steps to eliminate it. I believe that that is why I am now so much better. Let me hypothesise. Lead is a cumulative poison; let us suppose that aluminium is also. The disease is characterised by a very slow progression.

A thought has occurred to me. I wonder if Alzheimer's disease is misnamed. Could it be that it is not a disease at all, but the body's reaction to aluminium or mercury poisoning? Perhaps the steady degeneration of its victims is not an indication of the progress of a disease, but merely the result of a steady and continuous build-up of a cumulative metallic poison. I would be interested to hear of any research being done to ensure that a victim is not ingesting further quantities of these metals that then noted a slowing or halting of their symptoms.

I believe that the connection with aluminium or mercury (that the medical world seems to disagree about) exists. I once saw a graph showing the increase of Alzheimer's disease cases in this century, overlaid on a similar graph on the increased use of aluminium, and another on the increased use of amalgam dental fillings. Unfortunately, I cannot remember where I saw it, so if any readers come across a similar one, I would be grateful if they would send me a copy. I intend to write a further book on Alzheimer's disease, and would welcome any other feedback from readers.

Is there any action I would recommend to a victim of Alzheimer's disease or their carer? Yes, first, get rid of any medicines, cooking utensils, containers or wrapping material containing aluminium. I would recommend this to anyone, as we are all potential victims. Personally, I no longer frequent restaurants or hotels as I used to, as they normally use aluminium cookware.

I would recommend magnesium, contained in such things as multivitamin capsules, to help eliminate any aluminium at present in the body. (Health food shops sell a product called Silicol that is rich in magnesium.)

In Dr Michael A. Weiner's book Reducing the Risk of Alzheimer's, he mentions that lecithin contains phosphatidyl choline, and that, I quote, 'Any agent that could increase the quantity of acetylcholine in the brain would be of great benefit in the treatment of Alzheimer's disease and other senile dementias.' He lists the foods that contain lecithin. These are egg yolks, brewer's yeast, soyabeans, fish, beef liver, peanuts, wheat germ and whole grains. I have made sure that my diet contains plenty of magnesium and lecithin and perhaps this is another reason for my improvement.

The mental therapy I practised may not be suitable for many people; it may not, in any case, have played a part in my recovery.

I now have no symptoms of the disease. The procedures I took to combat it were rigorous and exhausting. I doubt whether I could do them again. A symptom of the disease is a diminishment of mental ability, energy and determination. It is doubtful whether I could have carried them out if I had not begun before the disease had gained too much of a hold.

The possibility exists that I did not have the disease in the first place. Perhaps all the doctors were wrong. I do not place much credence on this.

Let the reader be the judge, but above all do not give up hope. Everyone you speak to will tell you that there is no hope once you are diagnosed as having Alzheimer's disease. THEY ARE WRONG! There is always hope. I believe that I have had Alzheimer's disease and that I have recovered. If I am right then there is hope for others.

If I am wrong, and I was incorrectly diagnosed and never had Alzheimer's disease at all, then there is still hope for others: the hope that their own diagnosis will eventually be proved to be incorrect. I had all the usual symptoms, and all the necessary tests were undertaken to eliminate other causes. Although a firm diagnosis of Alzheimer's disease cannot be made until after the victim's death, the conclusion must be made that if I was mis-diagnosed, then so may many others be.

They say a traumatic experience can trigger the disease.

By far the most traumatic experience I have ever experienced was being told I had it and that there was no cure.

If I was misdiagnosed, then how many other patients are living out their lives under a similar misapprehension? If convinced that they have the disease, they will probably continue to to exhibit the symptoms needlessly. However, if given the slightest hope that there may be a cure, or that they may have been misdiagnosed, they will have something to live for and may well recover.

Incidentally, several nurses and other members of staff of nursing homes have told me that they suspect that a number of the Alzheimer's patients in their care do not have the disease. However, as the medical profession is adamant that there is no known cure, the only way such patients will be re-classified is for the doctor to admit that the initial diagnosis was false, and this they are naturally reluctant to do.

ALUMINIUM

Aluminium is by far the most abundant metal on earth. It makes up 8 per cent of the Earth's crust. of all the elements, only oxygen (47 per cent) and silicon (28 per cent) exceed it. It has a very strong affinity to oxygen, which explains why it withstood all attempts to prepare it in its elemental form until the 1880s. It was not commercially available until 1888 when the Bayer Process of separating aluminium from the bauxite ore was patented.

It has been used for the manufacture of pots, pans and other food preparation items at a progressive rate since the beginning of this century and today the packaging industry is by far the largest user of aluminium. Much of it is used in the production of drink containers, and a fair proportion of the drinks are of the fizzy, acidic type.

Alois Alzheimer first observed a physical cause of dementia in 1903. He published his findings in 1906 when he described the changes in a woman's brain that became known as Alzheimer's disease.

A progressive rate has occurred in the incidence of Alzheimer's disease since its discovery. In fact the increasing number of cases of Alzheimer's disease has almost paralleled the increased usage of aluminium.

Post-mortems of people with Alzheimer's disease have found high concentrations of aluminium salts in the brain cells. When the plaques that cover the brains of Alzheimer's disease victims were dissected, they invariably contained a few molecules of aluminium at the centre.

Although aluminium is ingested through food and water, in normally healthy people most of it is usually excreted. However, in a small percentage of people, with perhaps a weakened blood-brain barrier membrane, it remains in the body and is allowed to reach the brain.

In scientific tests aluminium has caused brain tangles and memory loss when injected into animals. The tangles are similar to the neurofibrillary tangles in Alzheimer's disease.

Scientists in Cambridge's 'Brain Bank Laboratory' have discovered that aluminium causes changes in the brain's tau. Tau is a protein essential for a healthy brain to maintain the neurological pathways. The changes they discovered were similar to the changes reported in post-mortems of Alzheimer's disease victims.

Recently some kidney patients undergoing dialysis suffered a form of dementia similar to Alzheimer's disease. Aluminium was found in the dialysis fluid, and when it was removed, the incidence of dementia was halted.

In January 1989 the Lancet published an article showing a relationship between the aluminium content in the drinking water and the extent of Alzheimer's disease developing in people under 70. This was carried out in 88 districts of England and Wales. The study showed that the risk of Alzheimer's disease was 150 per cent higher in districts where the concentration of aluminium in drinking water was more than ten times higher than average.

I think that it would be wise for everyone to ensure that they do not poison themselves with aluminium, and perhaps chelate out any aluminium that they may have absorbed.

As I have already said, get rid of any medicines, cooking utensils, containers or wrapping material containing aluminium. Do not drink acidic drinks such as cola from aluminium cans. Do not wrap meat or poultry in aluminium foil prior to cooking it in the oven. I believe that the high temperature combined with fat and juices splashing on to the foil may cause molecules of aluminium to migrate on to the food. Do not take stomach remedies or other medication containing aluminium, unless your doctor prescribes it to alleviate a more serious condition. (Offhand, I cannot think of one.) Beware of deodorants that contain aluminium as I believe that it may migrate through the pores of the skin in the sensitive areas to which these deodorants are usually applied. Campaign vigorously to stop your local water board adding aluminium to your domestic water supply. Most people are unaware that water authorities use a toxic metal, aluminium, to 'purify' the water. As the accumulation of aluminium seems to be hastened if there is a calcium deficiency – apparently the blood taking in aluminium in place of the missing calcium – I would recommend an adequate supply of dairy products.

There are medical methods of chelating aluminium from the brain but the following natural foods containing sulphur, listed in the previously mentioned book by Dr Weiner, perform almost as well: onions, garlic, chives, red pepper and egg yolks. They will also remove other heavy metal poisons such as lead and cadmium.

As well as ensuring that I was not ingesting any aluminium, I ate large quantities of these sulphur-containing foods, and that alone could be the reason for my improvement.

Incidentally, there is a simple test to determine whether there is excess aluminium in the body. This is by hair analysis and can be ordered through your doctor. It is known by the somewhat long-winded title of 'flameless atomic absorption analysis of acid-digested hair samples'.

Magnesium, contained in such things as multivitamin capsules, will also help to eliminate any aluminium at present in the body. (As I have said already, health food shops sell a product called Silicol that is rich in magnesium.)

Lecithin contains phosphatidyl choline, and any agent that could increase the quantity of acetylcholine in the brain would be of great benefit in the treatment of Alzheimer's disease and other senile dementias. As I said above, the foods that contain lecithin are egg yolks, brewer's yeast, soyabeans, fish, beef liver, peanuts, wheat germ and whole grains. I made sure that my diet contained plenty of magnesium and lecithin and I believe that this may have contributed to my recovery.

MERCURY

As I have said, I now consider mercury to be the worst culprit of all. I am hoping to be able to research this further. At present the following facts may be helpful.

There is strong evidence that mercury damages the brain and this metal is linked to Alzheimer's disease in several journals. Never allow your dentist to use amalgam (whose major constituent is mercury) as a dental filling material. If you already have amalgam fillings it is better, although disquieting, to leave them in situ rather than have them removed or replaced with enamel, as the process of drilling them out can itself produce mercury vapours that may migrate to the brain. However, if you are in the habit of grinding your teeth, and these contain amalgam fillings, it is probably better to take the risk of having the fillings drilled out, rather than constantly being exposed to the mercury vapours given off when the amalgam is disturbed. There is a halfway measure I have adopted, and that is to have the fillings crowned with white enamel. This may also require a certain amount of drilling, but not as much as complete removal of the amalgam. Children are more at risk from amalgam fillings than adults, simply because they are likely to have them for a longer period, so in their case I would think that it is probably better to have the fillings removed and replaced with enamel. It is a difficult decision that should be considered separately in each individual case.

I now study the ingredients on labelled food far more diligently than before, and occasionally I am horrified at what I find they contain. Take Cadbury's chocolates, for instance. I looked at the list of ingredients on their box after I had eaten a couple of chocolates and at the bottom was the word cochineal. I wish I had looked sooner, as I was aware that cochineal is derived from the cochineal beetle. However, I also recalled from my research that it had some connection with aluminium, but as I could not recall the precise details I wrote to Cadbury's for further information. I must say that they were very helpful in supplying the information I asked for, but on reading their reply, I was even more disturbed at having eaten the chocolates than before. An extract from their letter reads:

> 'The term Cochineal covers two products, one of which is soluble. Both products contain aluminium complexes of carminic acid. It is not permitted in the diets of Jehovah's Witnesses, Vegetarians, Jews and Vegans.

The process involves harvesting of the female beetle, just before egg laying commences and drying, washing at 90°C to remove any insect fragments, then reacting with aluminium at 95°C.

Cochineal is an approved colour and is safe and sterile. While these facts make cochineal an acceptable ingredient for the vast majority of consumers, I can nevertheless understand that you may have personal objections to eating food containing cochineal.'

I am amazed at both the frankness of Cadbury's reply and their naïevty in believing that consumers feel it is acceptable to use beetles as an ingredient of their chocolate. I believe that the only reason most consumers find it acceptable is that they are not aware of the nature of the product.

*   *   *

Finally, I would like to say that I may have appeared something of a braggart in the story, but it was necessary to show the reader how much I had deteriorated. I apologise for this as I consider myself a modest, unassuming sort of chap.

Sylvia says that she is glad somebody does.

*   *   *

And that was supposed to be the end of my story.

The manuscript had been written, had a second and third draft, a final polish, and was ready to send to a publisher.

Then I read a book that I wish I had not. It was a well-written book, and it is through no fault of the author that I wish I had never set eyes on it. The book, Alzheimer's – Caring for Your Loved One, *by Sharon Fish had an article near the end that disturbed me deeply, and made me re-evaluate my actions since I was first diagnosed as having the disease.*

This article Sharon Fish herself has taken from another book whose author was an Alzheimer's disease sufferer. He is Robert Davis, a Presbyterian minister. I quote from his book My Journey into Alzheimer's:

'I go to church services to worship God, but I cannot sing. I cannot join the reading or prayers because my mind cannot do two things at once. Singing and group readings take several processes going on at once to listen to the others and pace my reading in time with theirs. Such a simple thing. But impossible for me now.

Suddenly, I stand out in the worship service, silent and continually confused during the time of hymn singing. I feel that my fellow worshippers are looking at me askance, wondering why I do not join in. My new found paranoia also sets in, making me wonder if they think by my silence I am showing disapproval of the hymn, the church, the musicians, or the people around me. This time of joy has been changed into a time of frustration and anxiety.

Now, I would like to come into the service late, after the singing of the first hymn, or any responsive reading. However, out of propriety, I do not. How I long to again sing my heart out and thus fully express my joy, but I cannot. The sorrow of this and this sense of loss fills me so much that often tears come to my eyes – tears that only compound my paranoia and my ever-present fears of what people are thinking.

In my rational moments, I am still me.

Alzheimer's disease is like a reverse ageing process. Having drunk from the fountain of youth, one is caught in the time tunnel without a stopping place at the height of beauty and strength. Cruelly, it whips us back to the place of infancy. First the memories go, then perception, feelings, knowledge, and, in the last stage, our ability to talk and take care of our most basic human needs. Thrusting us headlong into the seventh age of man, "without teeth, without sight, without everything".

At this stage, while I still have control of thoughts and feelings, I must learn to take on the role of the infant in order to make use of whatever gifts are left to me.'

They are wonderful words, well written and full of meaning. However, they told me nothing that I did not already know. It was not what Robert Davis had written that disturbed me. It was the fact that he was able to write it.

I suddenly realised why I had written this book. It was not for the normal reason that I wanted it published for others to read. Admittedly, that is the reason I THOUGHT I was writing it, but I now see that I was deluding myself.

No, the reason I was writing it was to prove to myself that I did not have the disease. I did not believe that a person with such an illness could write a book like this. Now I see that I am wrong. The prose of Robert Davis has proved it to me.

One of the symptoms of Alzheimer's disease is self-delusion. The sufferers will not admit that they have it. And is not my so-called cure perhaps just such a delusion?

Could there be anything worse than having Alzheimer's disease?

Yes, for me there could. The one thing that would be worse than having the disease would be KNOWING that I have it.

I feel like a swimmer in an endless ocean, with the thought that the tide of fog may soon be coming in to drown my mind again.

Will it ever recede?

I try to think of something else.

* * *

Since the completion of this book two years ago, there has been no deterioration in my condition.

Author's Note

*

After I recovered from my illness, I wrote this book as a limited edition, bound it myself, and distributed it to a few close friends and relatives. When asked to release it for general distribution, I hesitated. Perhaps the treatment I undertook would work as well for others as I believed it had for me. Or perhaps not. If not, it may bring a sense of false hope to an Alzheimer's disease sufferer or to their relatives, who may read my book as avidly as a drowning man clutches at a straw.

I decided to go ahead anyway. When I was diagnosed as having Alzheimer's disease, I was in a black pit of total despair. I sought hope and solace from books, but there was none to be had. Any hope, false or otherwise, would have been welcome to me, and may have lifted my spirits a fraction.

If this book can raise the spirits of a victim or their carers for a few moments, I will feel rewarded for the work I have put into it. And if I saw a drowning man clutching at a straw, I would not jump in and take away the straw.

Louis Blank